PROBLEMS
IN THE RHEUMATIC DISEASES

Lessons from Patients

PROBLEMS IN THE RHEUMATIC DISEASES

Lessons from Patients

Ronald A Asherson, MD, FACP, FCP(SA)

Stephen H Morgan MB, MRCP

and Graham R V Hughes, MD, FRCP

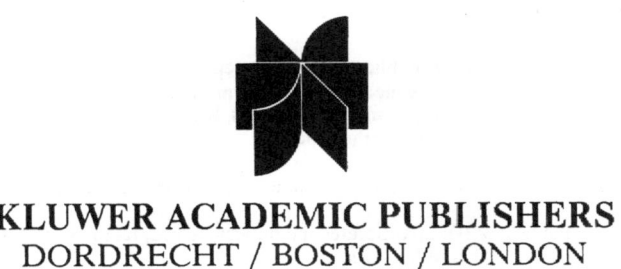

KLUWER ACADEMIC PUBLISHERS

DORDRECHT / BOSTON / LONDON

Distributors

for the United States and Canada: Kluwer Academic Publishers, PO Box 358, Accord Station, Hingham, MA 02018-0358, USA
for all other countries: Kluwer Academic Publishers Group, Distribution Center, PO Box 322, 3300 AH Dordrecht, The Netherlands

British Library Cataloguing in Publication Data

Asherson, R. A.
    Problems in the rheumatic diseases.
    1. Connective tissues – Diseases
    I. Title II. Morgan, S. III. Hughes, G.
    616.7'7   RC924

    ISBN-13:978-94-010-7050-8   e-ISBN-13:978-94-009-1241-0
    DOI:10.1007/978-94-009-1241-0

Library of Congress Cataloging in Publication Data

Asherson, R. A. (Ronald)
    Problems in the rheumatic diseases.

    Includes bibliographies and index.
    1. Connective tissues – Diseases. I. Morgan, S. (Stephen)
II. Hughes, Graham R. V. (Graham Robert Vivian) III. Title.
[DNLM: 1. Connective Tissue Diseases – diagnosis. 2. Connective
Tissue Diseases – therapy. WD 375 A825d]
RC924.A84 1988   616.7'7   87-17096
ISBN-13:978-94-010-7050-8

CONTENTS

v

CONTENTS

INTRODUCTION

Any physician travelling to other centres throughout the world must be struck by the similarity of the problems in diagnosis and management faced by fellow colleagues in rheumatology.

Despite the international spread of journals and of standard textbooks, the same practical questions constantly appear – how do you manage the psychotic patient with cerebral lupus, or the patient with intractable polymyositis, or the rheumatoid patient who has failed on almost all known therapeutic agents. Is it worth differentiating various 'overlap' syndromes? How can one improve on the classification and treatment of vasculitis?

Two questions – what is the patient telling us? and what can we do for the patient? are always central to the discussion.

Although these high-minded ideals are often not fulfilled, frequently something new appears to come from individual case presentations. These cases, discussed at our weekly conferences, were contributed by a number of different staff members. Where possible, a standard format has been use in each case presentation and a comment added where indicated. A short list of relevant references has been included with each case.

The aim of this book is to provide examples of these clinical problems and our own clinical approach to them – sometimes successful, sometimes not.

G R V Hughes,
Head, Lupus-Arthritis Research Unit,
The Rayne Institute,
St Thomas' Hospital,
London

ACKNOWLEDGEMENTS

We would like to acknowledge the contributions of our colleagues, listed here, in compiling the case reports:

- Elaine Baguley, MB MRCP, ARC Research Fellow, The Rayne Institute, St Thomas' Hospital, London

- Robert M Bernstein, MD MRCP, Consultant Rheumatologist, Manchester Royal Infirmary, Manchester

- Christopher C Bunn, PhD, Senior Technician, Rheumatology Unit, Department of Medicine, Royal Postgraduate Medical School, London

- Joel David, MB MRCP, Senior Registrar, Rheumatology Unit, Hammersmith Hospital, London

- Helen J Englert, FRACP, Research Fellow, Institute of Tropical Diseases, London

- Charlotte Feldman, FRCP, Consultant Rheumatologist, King Edward Hospital, Ealing, London

- Edward Gordon-Smith, FRCS, Professor of Haematology, St George's Hospital, London

- Lawrence Hart, MD, Rheumatology Fellow, McMaster University, Canada

- Richard G Hull, MB MRCP, Senior Registrar, Rheumatology, Wexham Park Hospital, Slough, Bucks

- Robin P Kennett, BSc MB MRCP, Research Fellow, Institute of Neurology, London

- Peter J Long, MB ChB DPhys Med, Senior Specialist in Rheumatology, Royal Air Force, and Clinical Assistant, Rheumatology Unit, St Thomas' Hospital, London

- Charles G Mackworth-Young, MA MD MRCP, Senior Registrar, Rheumatology Unit, Hammersmith Hospital, London

– Roger Reynolds, FRACP, Visiting Fellow, Rheumatology Unit,
  Department of Medicine, Royal Postgraduate Medical School, London

– Martin Ridley, MB MRCP, Senior Registrar, Rheumatology Unit,
  St Thomas' Hospital, London

– Carey Wolfe, MB MA MRCP, Registrar, Rheumatology Unit,
  St Thomas' Hospital, London

We also thank Dr R W E Watts (Consultant Physician, Northwick Park
Hospital, Middlesex) for allowing us to include cases 6.1 and 8.2.

Section 1

SYSTEMIC LUPUS ERYTHEMATOSUS AND RELATED DISORDERS

INTRODUCTION

At times the gulf between laboratory and clinical interests in SLE seems wide. In any conference on recent trends in lupus, the concentration of interest on one side of this divide is on blotting techniques, receptor kinetics and chromosome mapping, and, on the other, management of CNS lupus, the thrombosis – antiphospholipid syndrome, and pulse immunosuppressive regimes.

Yet in few other diseases have scientific advances made such obvious inroads into clinical management. Certainly, the treatment of SLE is still largely based on steroids and 'clinical judgement'. However, the enormously improved survival figures in the past decade surely reflect at least some of these advances, in addition to the clinical recognition of milder cases.

Epidemiology

SLE is now a major disease worldwide. Figures from the Americas, Asia and China, and the Caribbean give prevalence figures of up to 1 in 1000. There is a remarkable homogeneneity in the age and sex data (females outnumbering males by 9:1). Indeed, in view of recent HLA associations, it is perhaps surprising that the prevalence figures do not differ more widely. Perhaps in some south-east Asian countries, where the disease is prevalent, the figures will increase as socio-economic change brings in milder cases.

Clinical features

Some clinical features of lupus – the migraines, transient psychiatric disorders, recurrent spontaneous abortions, and the neonatal syndromes, have been highlighted in the past decade and are discussed in this chapter.

From the author's point of view, the topic which has exercised us most has been the antiphospholipid antibody syndrome. This syndrome, highlighted by our unit during the past 5 – 10 years, includes recurrent thrombosis, recurrent intrauterine deaths and cerebral disease (frequently strokes). The syndrome may also include thrombocytopaenia, livedo reticularis, chorea, myelopathy and labile hypertension. The development of immunoassays for anti-phospholipid antibodies, such as those directed against cardiolipin, has provided a new perspective on the aetiology of thrombosis in more general

2

terms, and increasing numbers of non-SLE patients with 'idiopathic' recurrent thrombosis, strokes, DVTs, Budd–Chiari syndrome, etc. are now being described in association with these antibodies.

Immunology

In addition to the clinically important antiphospholipid antibodies, considerable advances have been made into the definition, by blotting and other techniques, of some of the numerous antigen–antibody systems in SLE. Many of the antigens, such as Jo-1, RNP, Ro, etc. have been clinically identified, and the clinical relevance of anti-'ENA' antibodies more clearly defined. Thus anti-Ro is associated with photosensitive skin rashes and sometimes with ANA-negativity, and occasionally with congenital heart block; anti-RNP is associated with Raynaud's; and anti-Sm may be more prevalent in certain ethnic groups.

Aetiology

The finding of a C4 null allele in the majority of SLE patients and also the HLA Dr 3 association has given support for a basic genetically-determined defect in this disease.

Animal studies providing indirect evidence of viral triggering factors have, as yet, not been confirmed directly in humans. Other influences on the disease are sex hormones, and their possible relevance to therapy are touched on in the case discussions in this book.

Management

Immunosuppressive therapy, notably 'pulse' IV cyclophosphamide, has now become an accepted part of the management of severe SLE. While corticosteroids remain the mainstay of treatment, the high cost of aseptic necrosis of joints and of opportunistic infections has become more appreciated. The use of antimalarial therapy in SLE has broadened from its previous restriction to skin and joint disease. Idiosyncratic reactions to certain drugs, such as the hepatotoxicity sometimes seen with high-dose aspirin, are better recognized.

Treatments still included in the 'experimental' category include plasmapheresis, modulation with sex hormones and anticoagulation.

Perhaps the most significant advance in the management of SLE during the past two decades has been the general move to more conservative treatment – a reflection of the realization that, in the majority of patients, the ultimate prognosis is good. Credit for education in modern attitudes to treatment must go as much to patients and their 'self help' groups as to the physicians looking after them.

Further reading

1. Hughes G R V. Systemic lupus erythematosus. *Clin. Rheum. Dis.* 1982: **8**, 1
2. Lahita R. *Systemic Lupus Erythematosus.* (Chichester: Wiley) 1987

1.1   SEX AND SYSTEMIC LUPUS ERYTHEMATOSUS

History

Mr I.D., a gardener, first presented to his general practitioner with a scaly facial rash and a cough productive of green sputum. He was given antibiotics but returned two weeks later with extension of the rash to his trunk, and painful mouth ulcers. He was referred as a matter or urgency to his local hospital and found to have proteinuria and abnormal biochemical renal function (urea 18.7 mmol/L, creatinine 204 mcmol/L). Prednisolone 60 mg daily was started, and, although his rash improved, his renal function continued to deteriorate and he was referred for further investigations and treatment.

Examination revealed a widespread blistering rash and digital infarcts, as well as severe aphthous ulceration of the mouth. Surprisingly he had clinical dextrocardia (confirmed by chest X-ray).

Investigations

Hb	10.6 g/dl
WC	4.7×10^9/L (lymphopaenic)
ESR	104 mm/h
Urea	21.6 mmol/L
Creatinine	280 mcmol/L
Creatinine clearance	85 ml/min
Proteinuria	2.0 g/24 h
Urinary sediment	active

His ANA was positive at 1:640 with DNA binding of 95% and negative ENA. He had detectable cryoglobulinaemia.

Progress and management

Prednisolone was continued at a dose of 60 mg daily and azathioprine introduced. His renal function improved and the DNA binding fell to 50%. He became increasingly depressed and a week after admission attempted suicide by jumping from a second floor window sustaining fractures of pelvis and skull, and rupture of his spleen. At laparotomy for splenectomy, normal visceral anatomy was demonstrated. His stay on intensive care was complicated by bronchopneumonia, septicaemia and a period of acute tubular necrosis. His immunosuppression was continued and he eventually made a good recovery with return of mental and renal function to normal.

Points for discussion

A diagnosis of SLE was made on the basis of his rash, renal disease and abnormal serology. He had several mucocutaneous manifestations of SLE, including aphthous ulcers, a scaly rash and digital vasculitis.

SLE is relatively rare in men, the female to male ratio being 9:1. High levels of oestrogen appear to favour the development of SLE and its persistence, although low levels of testosterone found in male patients are probably not a predisposing risk factor.

Dextrocardia was a further interesting finding in this patient. Although there were no other detectable genetic abnormalities, the coexistence of SLE with other developmental abnormalities such as Kleinfelter's syndrome has been described.

Neuropsychiatric manifestations of SLE, once thought rare, are now recognized as increasingly common, occurring in at least 50% of patients. Differentiation between lupus cerebritis and steroid psychosis continues to remain a dilemma, no useful imaging techniques being of any help.

Comment

Steroid psychosis is very rare. Psychosis in SLE is common. In an SLE patient developing psychosis, a trial of corticosteroid therapy (up to 60 mg daily) for a week or two is worthwhile.

References

1. Dubois E L. *Lupus Erythematosus*. (University of California Press) 1974: 232–242
2. Mackworth-Young C G, Parke A L, Morley K D, Fotherby K and Hughes G R V. Sex hormones in male patients with SLE and other chronic diseases. *Eur. J. Rheumatol. Inflamm.* 1983: 6, 228–232
3. Estes D and Christian C L. The natural history of SLE by prospective analysis. *Medicine* 1971: 50, 85–100
4. Lahita R G. Sex steroids and the rheumatic diseases. *Arthritis Rheum.* 1985: 28, 121–125
5. Ortiz-Nels C, LeRoy E C. The co-incidence of Kleinfelter's syndrome and systemic lupus erythematosus. *Arthritis Rheum.* 1969: 12, 241–246

1.2   ACUTE CEREBRAL DISEASE – A DIFFICULT DIAGNOSIS

History

T.R., an 18-year-old clerk, first became unwell in 1982 with fever, arthralgia, pleurisy and microscopic haematuria. SLE with nephritis was diagnosed and her symptoms subsided on 30 mg prednisolone daily. Two years later she was admitted as an emergency in status epilepticus. Many features of active disease were obvious on examination, including mucosal ulcers, alopecia and cutaneous vasculitis, and examination of her urinary sediment suggested persisting glomerulonephritis. Her blood pressure was 180/130 mmHg and she had several further generalized tonic–clonic seizures during the first few days after admission. In between these she remained deeply unconscious, although with no focal neurological signs evident. Fundoscopy revealed tortuous vessels and a few retinal haemorrhages, but no papilloedema.

Investigations

Hb	8.6 g/dl. Normochromic normocytic
WC	6.5×10^9/L
Urea	11.0 mmol/L
Creatinine	143 mcmol/L
ANA	1:640, homogenous pattern
DNA binding	98%
ECG	sinus rhythm. LVH
EEG	excess intermediate slow wave activity with no focal features

Progress and management

Chlormethiazole was initially given to control the seizures, followed by intravenous phenytoin. Despite control of the seizures, there were dramatic fluctuations in her level of consciousness, with stupor or coma developing when the diastolic blood pressure exceeded 120 mmHg. When this was controlled with intravenous sodium nitroprusside, she became alert and communicative. High-dose prednisolone and cyclophosphamide were used to suppress disease activity.

Points for discussion

During acute 'flares' of SLE, the cause of a depressed level of consciousness can present a difficult diagnostic problem. In this patient, an initial diagnosis of hypertensive encephalopathy complicating her nephritis was made, although, equally, the fluctuations in blood pressure may have been due to 'cerebral lupus' causing central abnormalities of homeostatic control.

Convulsions accompanying hypertension in SLE carry a poor prognosis and treatment should be directed at:

1. Correction of hypertension with intravenous sodium nitroprusside or labetalol;
2. Control of seizures as described;
3. Immunosuppression of the underlying SLE. 'Pulsed' cyclophosphamide (500 mg – 1 g) is probably the most effective immediate method of achieving this today.

Comment

This case demonstrates that in the sick SLE patient, a variety of potentially treatable factors may contribute to convulsions.

References

1. Bennett R N, Hughes G R V, Bywaters E G L and Holt J P C. Neuropsychiatric problems in SLE. *Br. Med. J.* 1972: **4**, 342–344
2. Sergent J S, Lockshin M C, Klempner M S and Lipsey J A. Central nervous system disease in SLE. *Am. J. Med.* 1975: **58**, 644–654
3. Hughes, G R V. Central nervous system lupus – diagnosis and treatment. *J. Rheumatol.*, 1980: **7**, 405–411
4. Harris E N, Hughes, G R V. Cerebral disease in systemic lupus erythematosus. *Springer Semin. Immunopathol.* 1985: **8**, 251–266

1.3   DRUG-INDUCED LUPUS

History

A 52-year-old woman presented to her general practitioner with diastolic hypertension. She was initially treated with atenolol, and subsequently hydralazine at a dose of 50 mg qds was added. On this regimen smooth control of her hypertension was obtained.

A year later she noticed polyarthralgia and complained of chest pains which were pleuritic in character, and fevers.

Investigations

Hb	9.9 g/dl
WC	2.7×10^9/L
ESR	55 mm/h
ANA	positive 1:620, homogenous
DNA binding	18%
Immune complexes (C1q binding)	positive

A chest X-ray showed small bilateral pleural effusions.

Progress and management

The hydralazine was withdrawn and oral prednisolone introduced, with resolution of the clinical features. After two months the ESR had fallen to within normal limits and the ANA had become negative. Control of her hypertension was achieved by adding nifedipine.

Points for discussion

Drug-induced lupus is rare. Of the drugs implicated (Table 1.3), those used in the treatment of cardiovascular diseases predominate. A number of drugs may unmask or exacerbate existing SLE (penicillin, sulphonamides, oral contraceptives). The development of a positive ANA in patients taking hydralazine is dose related – occuring usually when the cumulative dose is greater than 200 g. Only a small percentage of these will develop a full-blown lupus syndrome, and CNS or renal involvement is unusual. Hydralazine induced lupus occurs almost invariably in slow acetylators and is common in HLA DR4 positive patients. Although the ANA (and LE cell test) may be strongly positive, high titres of anti-dsDNA are unusual. Although not routinely done, antibodies to ssDNA, and DNA-histone would be present in high titre. Remission following withdrawal of the drug may take several months.

Table 1.3 Drugs implicated in drug-induced LE

Cardiovascular drugs	Procainamide* Quinidine Practolol Hydralazine* Methyldopa Reserpine Captopril
Anticonvulsants	Phenytoin* Ethosuxamide Troxidone Primidone
Antimicrobials	Isoniazid* Griseofulvin Streptomycin
Others	Thiouracils Chlorpromazine* Penicillamine Phenylbutazone Methysergide

* most frequent

Comment

The frequency and importance of drug-induced lupus may have been overemphasized. In general, the finding of a positive ANA in a patient treated with the agents listed above is not a major threat.

References

1. Batchelor J R, Welsh K L, Tinoco R M *et al.* Hydralazine-induced SLE, the influence of HLA-DR and sex on suseptibility. *Lancet* 1980: 1, 1107–1109
2. Harman C E and Portanova J P. Drug-induced lupus: clinical and serological studies. *Clin. Rheum. Dis.* 1982: 8, 121–135
3. Bernstein R M, Egerton-Vernon J and Webster J. Hydralazine-induced cutaneous vasculitis. *Br. Med. J.* 1980: 208, 156–157

1.4   PANCYTOPAENIA

History

A 33-year-old woman had a four-year history of SLE. The major clinical manifestations being fever, polyarthritis, alopecia, malar rash, Raynaud's phenomenon and pleurisy. She had been treated with combinations of prednisolone and hydroxychloroquine (OHC) (Figure 1.4) and was on this occasion admitted from the out-patient department.

Investigations

Hb	7.6 g/dl	
WC	1.0×10^9/L –	neutrophils 66%
		lymphocytes 20%
		monocytes 9%
		metamyelocytes 5%
platelets	37×10^9/L	
ESR	85 mm/h	
DNA binding	50%	
Coombs' test	negative	

Progress and management

Antibodies to platelets and white cells were detectable. Bone marrow studies showed a normocellular marrow. Red cell survival studies were a third of normal (43 days) with marked splenic sequestration. The pancytopaenia was considered to be due to a combination of hypersplenism and active disease. The OHC was discontinued, she was given 3 x 1 g i.v. pulses of methylprednisolone, and the oral prednisolone increased to 60 mg/day (Figure 1.4). This resulted in a modest increase in WC and platelet count, but the haemoglobin continued to fall, necessitating red cell transfusions. Splenectomy was considered.

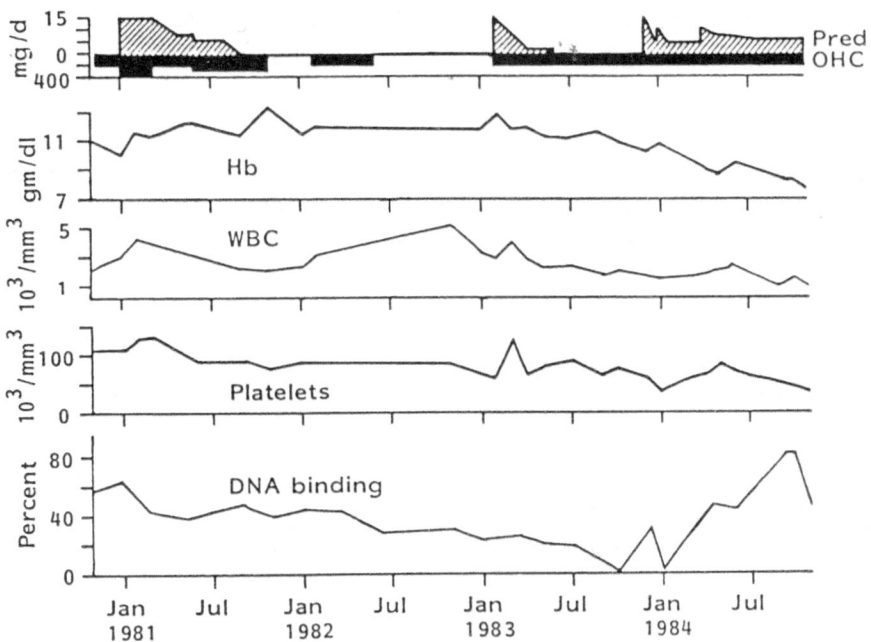

Figure 1.4 Response to treatment

Points for discussion

This is an extreme case of haematological and splenic involvement in systemic lupus erythematosus. Haematological abnormalities are very common in lupus and may involve red cells, white cells and platelets. Normochromic normocytic anaemia is the most common problem and is presumably due to retarded erythropoesis secondary to chronic inflammation. Haemolytic anaemia occurs in about 10% of patients and may be Coombs' positive or negative. Leukopaenia, particularly an absolute neutropaenia, is very common. Leukocytosis can occur and may be due to active lupus, steroid therapy, or infection. Mild thrombocytopaenia occurs in one third of lupus patients but only rarely do counts fall below 100 x 10^9/L.

Splenomegaly is present in 10–20% of patients, usually without haemolytic anaemia. The typical pathological finding of concentric periarterial fibrosis ('onion skin' lesions) may represent the result of a previous focal arteritis. Hypersplenism with pancytopaenia is rare. Splenectomy is occasionally required for control of thrombocytopaenia or anaemia. The

13

indications for this procedure in lupus, and its effect on the subsequent course of the disease, are unclear. Hyposplenism has also been reported.

Comment

If only we had an adequate test or tests which could help us in the common problem of leukopaenia in SLE – is it the disease or is it the azathioprine, for example, which the patient may have been taking?

References

1. Budman D R and Steinberg A D. Haematologic aspects of SLE. *Ann. Intern. Med.* 1977: **86**, 220 – 229
2. Rivero S J, Alger M and Alarcon-Segovia I. Splenectomy for haemocytopenia in SLE. *Arch. Intern. Med.* 1979: **139**, 773 – 776
3. Best W R and Starling D R. A critical look at the splenectomy – SLE controversy. A controlled appraisal. *Med. Clin. N. Am.* 1962: **46**, 19 – 47
4. Hall S, McCormick J L, Greipp P R, *et al.* Splenectomy does not cure the thrombocytopenia of systemic lupus erythematosus. *Ann. Intern. Med.* 1985: **102**, 325 – 328

1.5   MIGRAINOUS HEADACHES

History

A 29-year-old woman developed polyarthritis, principally affecting her wrists and the small joints of both hands. Since the age of 20, when she had had an unexplained episode of chorea, her history had been punctuated by two deep vein thromboses (DVT) and a pulmonary embolus. The second DVT occurred six weeks after the cessation of 6 months of warfarin therapy. She had also had two spontaneous abortions. She had complained of Raynaud's phenomenon for several years. On further questioning she admitted to several classical attacks of vertebrobasilar migraine over the previous year, with blurred vision, teichopsia, nausea and severe headache. She had also noticed attacks of paraesthesia in the limbs and gave a history of occasional vertigo. After one of these migrainous attacks she had developed a permanent left hemianopia.

Examination

Splinter haemorrhages on fingers. Marked livedo reticularis. Normotensive (BP 110/70 mmHg). All systems normal on clinical examination.

Investigations

Hb	12.0 g/dl
WCC	3.1×10^9/L
Platelets	49×10^9/L
ESR	90 mm/h
ANA	positive (1:40)
RA latex test	positive (1:40)
DNA binding	negative persistently
ENA	positive (anti-Ro)
Lupus anticoagulant	positive
Antibodies to cardiolipin	positive (IgG)
VDRL	negative
Immune complexes	absent
Schirmer's test	positive

Lip biopsy   normal
CT scan   cortical infarct present on right

Progress and management

The patient was diagnosed as having SLE, but although she was ANA and ENA positive, the DNA bindings were consistently negative, a finding present in up to 40% of our patients with the 'antiphospholipid syndrome' (APS), the disturbances accompanying her headaches were initially ascribed to migrainous phenomena, but in retrospect were probably transient ischaemic attacks (TIAs) which eventually resulted in a frank cerebral infarction. The migraines were severe and atypical and accompanied by thrombocytopenia, also a not uncommon finding in APS.

Our patient did not respond to prednisolone and pizotifen. She was eventually anticoagulated with warfarin and remains well.

Comment

In patients with frequent or complicated migraine, not responding to conventional therapy, this syndrome should be considered. It may occur in isolation or in association with 'frank' SLE. Formal anticoagulation should be considered to prevent cortical infarction.

Migraines are now recognized as one of the major features of SLE – and may antedate the diagnosis of SLE by many years. Fortunately, beta-blockers, used in many of these patients, rarely pose major problems in those lupus patients with mild Raynaud's.

The patient also demonstrates the phenomenon of 'recurrent' thrombosis following warfarin discontinuation which usually occurs 6–12 weeks after cessation of anticoagulation therapy in patients with high levels of anti-phospholipid antibodies.

References

1. Hughes G R V. Thrombosis, abortion, cerebral disease and the lupus anticoagulant. *Br. Med. J.* 1983: **287**, 1088–1089
2. Hughes G R V. The anticardiolipin syndrome. *Clin. Exp. Rheumatol.* 1985: **3**, 285–286
3. Editorial. Anticardiolipin antibodies, a risk factor for venous and arterial thrombosis. *Lancet* 1985: **1**, 912–913
4. Brandt K D and Lessell S. Migrainous phenomena in systemic lupus erythematosus. *Arthritis Rheum.* 1978: **21**,7–16

5. Isenberg D A, Meyrick-Thomas D, Snaith M L *et al.* A study of migraine in systemic lupus erythematosus. *Ann. Rheum. Dis.* 1982: **41**,30 – 32
6. Asherson R A and Harris E N. Anticardiolipin antibodies – clinical associations. *Postgrad. Med. J.* 1986: **62**, 1081 – 1087
7. Asherson R A, Chan J K H, Harris E N *et al.* Anticardiolipin antibody, recurrent thrombosis and warfarin withdrawal. *Ann. Rheum. Dis.* 1985: **44**, 823 – 825

1.6   ACUTE POLYRADICULONEUROPATHY

History

Over the past four years, a 58-year-old man had been treated with NSAIDs for an arthritis.

In 1985, he developed progressive weakness of his legs and tingling in the extremities and, over the next week, some weakness in the arms. He also complained of chest pain on deep inspiration.

At the time of referral he looked ill. There was a synovitis of the small joints of both hands and feet. There was marked facial diplegia, but no other bulbar signs. He had a flaccid and global weakness of all limbs. Similarly, the truncal muscles were too weak to overcome gravity. There was hypoaesthesia and hypoalgesia over the fingers and below the knees bilaterally. Position sensibility was impaired in the fingers and toes, and perception and vibration were lost below the anterior superior iliac spines. There was no evidence of sphincter or autonomic dysfunction.

Investigations

Hb	8.6 g/dl. normochromic normocytic
WC	normal
Platelets	114×10^9/L
ESR	108 mm/h
Urea	15.8 mmol/L
Creatinine	160 mcmol/L
Creatinine clearance	27 ml/min
Proteinuria	3.2 g/24 h
CRP	2.0 mmol g^{-1} ml^{-1}
ANA	positive 1:6400, homogenous pattern
DNA binding	normal
ENAs	not detected
Serum proteins	elevated (IgG = 21.4 G/L, IgM = 7.4 G/L)
Immune complexes (C1q binding, mRFBA)	positive
Cryoglobulins	positive

Serological tests for syphilis, hepatitis surface antigen and lupus anti-coagulant were all negative. Renal biopsy demonstrated a mesangio-proliferative glomerulonephritis with deposits of IgA, IgG, IgM and C3.

Nerve conduction studies: Small sensory action potential amplitudes, moderately slowed motor conduction velocity with delayed or absent F-waves. CSF: cellular, with an elevated protein content (1.09 g/L), and with oligoclonal IgG bands.

Progress and management

On the basis of the clinical picture, CSF protein and nerve conduction studies, a diagnosis of a Guillain–Barré type acute polyradiculoneuropathy was made. He also had features of a 'lupus-like' disease with glomerulo-nephritis despite normal DNA binding. He was initially treated with high-dose oral prednisolone, but because of clinical deterioration he was given 4 x 4 L plasma exchanges, a single intravenous pulse of 0.5 g cyclophosphamide and maintenance therapy was continued with oral azathioprine at a dosage of 50 mg tds.

Over the ensuing weeks he improved, with a fall in ESR and immuno-globulin levels. His renal function returned to normal and at discharge muscle power was in the MRC grade 4–4+ range.

Points for discussion

The Guillain–Barré syndrome is a predominantly motor neuropathy with areflexia and raised CSF protein. It is usually acute in onset. The eponym should be reserved for cases where the underlying aetiology is not known.

In one major review of 1100 cases an estimated cause for Guillain–Barré syndrome was found in 66%. Of these, less than 2% were related to a systemic connective tissue disease. This patient is also unusual in that he is male and developed SLE at a late age. It has been suggested that neurological complications are more common in this age group.

Although his disease features satisfy current ARA criteria for the classification of SLE, the DNA binding was normal. Again this appears to be characteristic of late-onset disease.

Comment

When we first described the various clinical associations of antiphospholipid antibodies, we wondered whether possible cross-reaction of these antibodies with CNS phospholipids might contribute directly to neurological disease. To date, we have little evidence for this from our studies.

References

1. Leneman F. The Guillain – Barré syndrome. *Arch. Intern. Med.* 1966: **118**, 139 – 144
2. McDonald D, Hutchinson M and Bresnihan B. The frequent occurence of neurologic disease in patients with late onset SLE. *Br. J. Rheumatol.* 1984: **23**, 186 – 189
3. Catoggio L J, Skinner R P, Smith G and Maddison P J. Systemic lupus erythematosus in the elderly, clinical and serological characteristics. *J. Rheumatol.* 1984: **11**, 175 – 181
4. Editorial. plasma exchange and neurological disorders. *Lancet* 1986: **2**, 1313 – 1314

1.7   SHRINKING LUNG SYNDROME

History

A 20-year-old girl working as a clerk presented in 1974 with fever, myalgias, joint pains, increased hairfall, Raynaud's syndrome, mouth ulcers and facial rash. The Schirmer's test of tear secretion was abnormally dry. DNA binding was elevated at 97% with a positive ANA, but the C3 complement level was normal. A diagnosis of systemic lupus erythematosus was made, and treatment with prednisolone and chloroquine was commenced.

In 1975, in addition to rash, fever and arthritis, she developed chest pain, breathlessness, tachypnoea and orthopnoea. The chest pain was persistent and dull, and was felt as a band around the lower chest. At times it was ascribed to pleurisy or pericarditis but friction rubs were never heard.

The ECG was normal and the chest radiograph showed raised diaphragms with patchy atalectasis in the lower zones (Figure 1.7). Ventilation and perfusion lung scanning showed no evidence of pulmonary embolism. Lung function tests showed a fall in vital capacity from 3.0 L (predicted normal 3.3) to 2.5 L over 3 months and then to 0.8 L over the following 5 months. The kCO or diffusion coefficient per unit of residual functional lung was maintained in the normal range at 1.85 – 1.95, and arterial blood gas tensions remained normal. The major finding was a severe loss of diaphragmatic muscle power measured as inspiratory pressure either across the diaphragm using gastric and oesophageal balloons, or more simply at the mouth with a hand-held barometer.

There was no evidence of generalized muscle weakness, and serum creatinine phosphokinase, a needle muscle biopsy and Tensilon test were all normal. A diagnosis of 'shrinking lung syndrome' was made.

Progress and management

Despite treatment which included oral prednisolone, azathioprine, cyclophosphamide and plasma exchange there was no improvement in her symptoms. She was only able to sleep at night with the help of a cuirasse respirator. Her hospital course was punctuated by a cardiac arrest complicating acute hyperkalaemia. She was resuscitated, and her condition became reasonably stable. Fearing the worst, her family took her home to Poland by car.

21

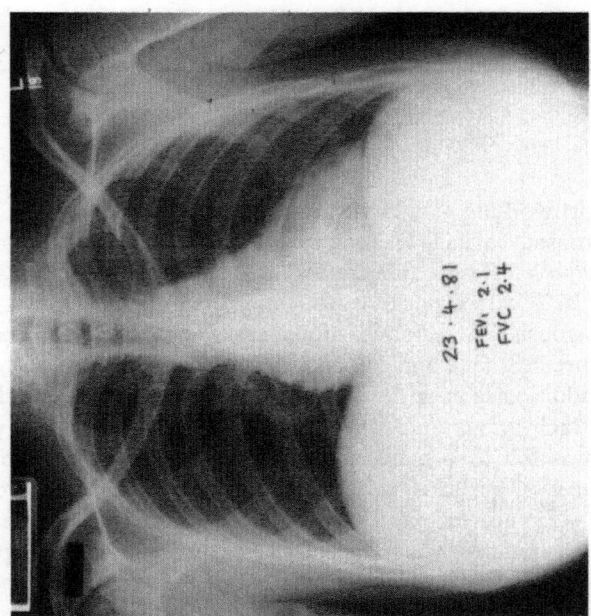
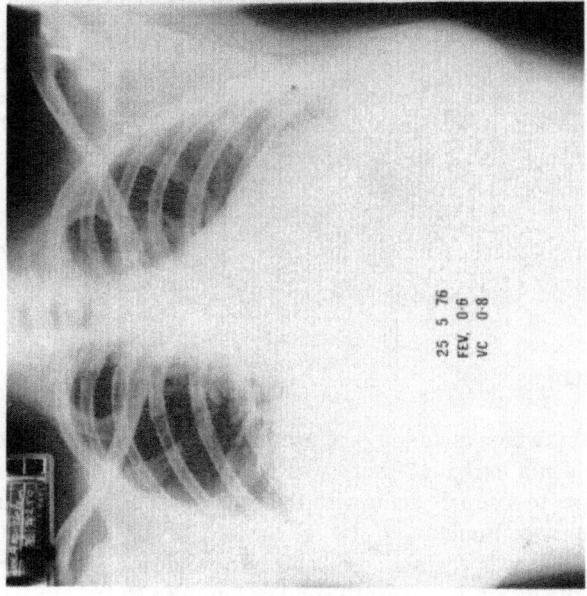

Figure 1.7 Shrinking lung syndrome. Chest radiographs before (left) and after (right) treatment

22

Three months later she returned feeling better with resolution of the fever and rash, and an increase in her vital capacity. She had, however, developed haemorrhagic cystitis on cyclophosphamide.

In 1979 all therapy was discontinued, but a year later the SLE flared and was again complicated by shrinking lung syndrome. Once again, treatment was aggressive, chlorambucil 5 mg daily being added. She steadily improved. Six years later, the chest X-ray and lung function are normal.

Points for discussion

Abnormalities of pulmonary function are common in SLE, but symptomatic dyspnoea is unusual and usually suggests pulmonary hypertension, thromboembolic disease, pulmonary fibrosis or shrinking lung syndrome.

Shrinking lung syndrome is characterized by band-like chest pain, dyspnoea, tachypnoea and orthopnoea, with small lung volumes and high diaphragms on chest X-ray. Arterial gas tensions are generally normal due to maintenance of a high minute volume to compensate for the proportionally increased anatomical dead space. The pathogenetic mechanism involves weakness of the diaphragm, hence dyspnoea is exacerbated by lying flat, as the abdominal viscera compress the lungs further.

Our case shows that shrinking lung syndrome is reversible although it is unclear whether immunosuppression therapy played a part in this. Among six of our patients followed with serial observations over 1–5 years, vital capacity on average doubled, and inspiratory pressure, reflecting strength of the diaphragm, tripled. Nevertheless, lung function may not return completely to normal, and the patient described above, after two episodes of shrinking lungs, has persistently elevated diaphragms and vital capacity less than half normal; however, she is not breathless at rest. One post mortem report noted fibrosis in the diaphragm. Thus it seems likely that the pathology is one of inflammation that resolves with scarring. This is primarily an extrapulmonary disease, and atelectatic changes in the lungs are secondary. The mechanism by which disease localizes in the diaphragm is unknown.

Comment

It is fortunate that this dramatic and highly characteristic pulmonary complication of SLE is very rare. Although we originally suggested that direct diaphragmatic involvement might contribute, 10 years later there is still very little data available on the pathophysiology of this condition.

References

1. Gibson G J, Edmonds J P and Hughes G R V. Diaphragm function and lung involvement in systemic lupus erythematosus. *Am. J. Med.* 1977: **63**, 926–932
2. Bernstein R M, Ind P W, Elkon K B, Sewell J R, Gibson G J, Hughes J M B and Hughes G R V. Pulmonary function in SLE with a longitudinal study of the shrinking lung syndrome. *Arthritis Rheum.* 1982: **25**, 56–60
3. Rubin L A and Urowitz M B. Shrinking lung syndrome in SLE; a clinical pathologic study. *J. Rheumatol.* 1984: **10**, 973–976

1.8   URTICARIAL VASCULITIS

History

A 53-year-old woman had first complained of recurrent fever, abdominal pains and diarrhoea at the age of 31. Nine years later she had an appendicectomy. The symptoms did not resolve and over the next 7 years she had two negative laparotomies. At 45 years she developed acute tenosynovitis and a polyarthritis. A discoid facial rash developed along with Raynauds's phenomenon, intermittent parotitis and Sicca syndrome. The year before she was referred to hospital, she had noticed a transient truncal rash which appeared urticarial, and was often associated with diarrhoea, and attacks of angio-oedema with swelling of the lips, periorbital oedema and acute dyspnoea.

Progress and management

Initial investigations were as shown:

Hb	10.4 g/dl
WC	$3.4 \times 10^9/L$
ANA	positive 1:2560 speckled pattern
DNA binding	<20%
ENAs	positive (anti-RNP)
Complement	low C4 levels (persistent)
C1q esterase levels	normal (quantitative and functional)

A working diagnosis of 'lupus-like' disease was made and oral steroids and azathioprine were started. The clinical response was poor. A skin biopsy showed features of a leukocytoclastic vasculitis, and dapsone and hydroxyzine were introduced, with some reduction in frequency of occurence of rash although not of angio-oedema. In view of the regularity with which the attacks occurred, a trial of plasmapheresis and pulsed i.v. cyclophosphamide was tried with only a partial improvement of her symptoms. Oral cromoglycate and transfusion of fresh frozen plasma were similarly disappointing.

Points for discussion

Although the clinical and serological features exhibited by this patient satisfy current ARA diagnostic criteria for SLE, her presentation is by no means classical and there were no detectable antibodies against double stranded DNA. Serologically, she would fulfil Sharp's criteria for a diagnosis of 'mixed connective tissue disease' with high titres of anti-RNP antibodies.

In the literature six similar patients with cutaneous vasculitis – urticaria – hypocomplementaemia syndrome are described. Two of these had high-titre ANAs with a speckled nuclear pattern although further characterization was not made.

The syndrome of hypocomplementaemic – urticarial vasculitis seems to affect women in their middle years, and is often associated with fever, abdominal pain, lymphadenopathy, and sometimes glomerulonephritis. 5 – 10% of patients with SLE may present with urticarial disease, and complement abnormalities are well described, although C1q levels are usually normal both quantitatively and functionally.

Comment

Treatment of this condition is most disappointing. Despite a variety of therapies, including steroids, immunosuppression, plasma exchange etc., the patient remained symptomatic and only self-administered steroid and adrenalin manage to avert life-threatening episodes of angio-oedema.

References

1. McDuffie F C, Sans W M, Maldonado P H, Conn D L and Sanayda E A. Hypocomplementaemia with cutaneous vasculitis and arthritis. *Mayo Clin. Proc.* 1973: **48**, 349 – 348
2. Sissons J G P, Gwynn Williams D, Peters D K and Boulton-Jones J M. Skin lesions, angio-oedema and hypocomplementaemia. *Lancet* 1974: **2**, 1350 – 1352
3. Monroe E W, Schultz C and Maize J. Vasculitis in chronic urticaria. *Clin. Res.* 1979: **27**, 713A
4. Gannon R W and Wheeler C E. Urticarial vasculitis. *Arch. Dermatol.* 1979: **115**, 76 – 80
5. O'loughlin S, Schroerer A L and Jordan R E. Chronic urticaria-like lesions in systemic lupus erythematosus. *Arch. Dermatol.* 1978: **63**, 485 – 490
6. Warin R P. Editorial. Urticarial vasculitis. *Br. Med. J.* 1983: **286**, 1919 – 1920

1.9   ISCHAEMIC COLON

History

A 44-year-old woman with a previous history of epilepsy had developed a polyarthritis just after the birth of her first child at the age of 26. A diagnosis of rheumatoid arthritis had been made and she had been treated with a combination of prednisolone and sodium aurothiomalate. In 1976, she developed a malar 'butterfly' rash, alopecia and Raynaud's phenomenon and complained of pleuritic chest pains. A clinical diagnosis of SLE was made and supported by a positive ANA and antibodies to double-stranded DNA. She was again treated with prednisolone, but developed a right hemiparesis a year later. This was attributed to cerebral vasculitis.

In 1980 she developed episodic abdominal pain and a diagnosis of subacute intestinal obstruction was made. On one occasion a laparotomy was performed and multiple peritoneal adhesions were resected. She developed proteinuria. Renal biopsy demonstrated a diffuse proliferative glomerulo-nephritis and azathioprine was added to her treatment.

A year later she was again admitted with peritonitis and features suggestive of ischaemic colitis.

Progress and management

A mesenteric angiogram confirmed obstruction of the coeliac axis with complete occlusion of the inferior mesenteric artery. A laparotomy was performed and the ischaemic bowel resected. A vascular graft was interposed between the aorta and hepatic and splenic arteries. Histologically the bowel showed features of ischaemic colitis, and the lumen of several arteries and veins were occluded by fresh or organizing thrombi. There were no inflammatory changes in the vessel walls and no histological features of vasculitis (Figure 1.9).

She made a good recovery but has since had a left leg deep vein thrombosis and numerous transient cerebral ischaemic episodes (TIAs). The partial thromboplastin time (PTT) was prolonged, although other clotting studies were normal. A circulating lupus anticoagulant was detected (LA), and, although VDRL was negative, anticardiolipin antibodies were present in high titre.

27

Points for discussion

The significance of LA, false positive serological tests for syphilis and anticardiolipin antibodies have been discussed in Case 1.5.

Although small vessel involvement is common in SLE, the involvement of large arteries is infrequently documented.

The gastrointestinal complications of SLE were first noted by Osler in 1895 and are now well recognized. Abdominal pain is the commonest symptom and this may be due to a number of factors, including acute pancreatitis and complications of treatment (peritonitis, peptic ulcer etc. Mesenteric vasculitis may produce mesenteric 'angina' or result in single or multiple perforations of the bowel.

In this patient, however, the pathological features were suggestive of primary *in situ* thrombosis leading to infarction. Since there was no evidence of vasculitis, this would suggest a pathogenic role for antiphospholipid antibodies in this patient's unusual disease course.

Comment

The term 'vasculitis' may have been used far too liberally in SLE. In some patients, the vascular pathology may be due to intimal disease and thrombosis rather than on an inflammatory basis.

References

1. Byron M A. The clotting defect in SLE. *Clin. Rheum. Dis.* 1982: **8**, 137–151
2. Alarcon-Segovia D and Osmundson P J. Peripheral vascular syndromes associated with SLE. *Ann. Intern. Med.* 1965: **62**, 907–919
3. Hoffman B I and Tata W A. The gastrointestinal manifestations of SLE. A review of the literature. *Semin. Arthritis Rheum.* 1980: **9**, 237–247
4. Zizic T M, Classen J N and Stevens M B. Acute abdominal complications of systemic lupus erythematosus and polyarteritic nodosa. *Am. J. Med.* 1982: **73**, 525–531

1.10   IDIOPATHIC PULMONARY HYPERTENSION AND DISCOID LE

History

In 1977 a 57-year-old woman presented with exertional syncope. These episodes became more frequent and she complained of increasing dyspnoea. There were no complaints of Raynaud's phenomenon. Three years later a diagnosis of idiopathic pulmonary hypertension was confirmed by right heart catheterization (mean pulmonary artery pressure of 64 mmHg). A pulmonary angiogram showed no evidence of thromboembolic disease, and CXR did not show pulmonary fibrosis. Nifedipine provided some symptomatic relief.

In 1982 she developed a rash over her sternum and knuckles which had the clinical and histological features of discoid lupus erythematosus and a small joint polyarthritis which was non-erosive and atypical in its distribution. She was admitted to hospital for evaluation.

Examination

Moderately obese; blood pressure 110/70 mmHg; no evidence of congestive failure; palpable second heart sound present; loud P_2 audible on auscultation; examination of RS, GIS and CNS essentially normal.

Investigations

FBC	normal
ESR	20 mm/h
RA latex test	negative
ANA	negative
DNA binding	negative
ENAs	negative
VDRL	positive (1:8). TPHA negative
Lupus anticoagulant	positive
Anticardiolipin antibodies	high positive (IgG, IgM)

Progress and managment

Her pulmonary hypertension steadily worsened with the mean pulmonary arterial pressure rising to 85 mmHg. The rash and arthritis were compatible with 'pure' discoid lupus. She was anticoagulated with warfarin and discharged once again on nifedipine, 20 mg bid.

Points for discussion

This patient clearly had DLE with no systemic or serological features to suggest SLE. False positive tests for syphilis sometimes occur in DLE, but their association with LA and anticardiolipin antibodies has not been described in DLE.

Pulmonary hypertension complicating SLE is uncommon but we have seen a number of such patients who have false positive serological tests for syphilis, LA and anticardiolipin antibodies, and have speculated about a causal link based on microthrombosis in pulmonary hypertension.

This patient represents an important link between pulmonary hypertension and the above triad of serological markers in that they were the only detectable immunological abnormalities present at the time of presentation.

Comment

This case makes the important point that discoid LE, despite its immunological 'blankness', may nevertheless demonstrate some of the features of systemic LE.

References

1. Asherson R A, Mackworth-Young C G, Boey M L, Hull R G, Saunders A E, Gharavi A E and Hughes G R V. Pulmonary hypertension in SLE. *Br. Med. J.* 1983: **287**, 1024–1025
2. Callen J P. Chronic cutaneous lupus erythematosus. *Arch. Dermatol.* 1982: **118**, 412–416
3. Asherson R A and Oakley C. Editorial. Pulmonary hypertension in systemic lupus erythenatosus. *J. Rheumatol.* 1986: **3**, 1–5
4. Asherson R A, Morgan S H, Harris E N *et al.* Pulmonary hypertension and chronic cutaneous lupus erythematosus: association with the lupus anticoagulant. *Arthritis Rheum.* 1985: **28**, 118

1.11 A CHINESE PUZZLE

History

Frances, a 30-year-old secretary, was of Chinese descent and first became ill after a holiday in Greece 3 years previously. Her face and arms became puffy and red following sun exposure, and on her return to England she developed a florid polyarthritis, painful mouth ulcers, pleurisy and alopecia. A clinical diagnosis of SLE was made and supported by serological findings. Proteinuria was detected and her urinary sediment suggested an active nephritis. She had a high fever.

She was given prednisolone 40 mg daily, but became psychotic and suicidal.

The combination of a high ESR and low CRP suggested that fever reflected active disease rather than intercurrent infection.

Investigations

Hb	12 g/dl
WC	3×10^9/L
Platelets	80×10^9/L
ESR	140 mm/h
ANA	positive
DNA binding	80%
CRP	1.0 mmol g^{-1} ml^{-1}

Progress and management

Three 1 g pulses of i.v. methylprednisolone were given and azathioprine was added to her existing treatment with prednisolone. The majority of her disease features improved – in particular the psychosis, but the fever persisted, as did her nephritis with a persistently 'active' urinary sediment and some deterioration in renal function. A renal biopsy confirmed an active lupus nephritis and two i.v. pulses of cyclophosphamide (0.5 g) were given. Her renal function improved, but the fever (38 – 39°C) continued and she became moderately short of breath. Although her CXR had previously been normal, a repeat film showed typical changes of miliary TB. Mycobacteria

31

were never isolated, but she improved dramatically on antituberculous chemotherapy.

Points for discussion

Fever in patients with SLE often causes a diagnostic puzzle, since active disease may produce a febrile response as easily as infection. The WC is often unhelpful, and, although it has been our experience that patients with SLE mount a moderate CRP response to infection rather than to active disease, this has not been a totally reliable indicator in our experience.

Infection is undoubtedly one of the principal contributory factors in mortality in SLE, and the frequency and range of infection in an unselected group of patients has been documented prospectively by Nived *et al*. In many cases the SLE was mild and the overall level of corticosteroid treatment low. There was a significant increase in bacterial infection rate irrespective of steroid dose, although no increased incidence of viral or fungal infections. *Staphylococcus aureus* was by far the most frequently implicated organism. Mycobacterium was only isolated in 1/58 patients, and opportunistic infection was rare and more often correlated with steroid treatment.

Comment

Tuberculosis continues to haunt the SLE patient.

References

1. Abeles M, Weinstein A and Aurier R B. Infections complicating the rheumatic diseases. In Grieco M N (ed.) *Infections in the Abnormal Host* 1980: (Yorke Medical Books)
2. Pepys M B, Lanham J G and DeBeer F C. C-reactive protein in SLE. *Clin. Rheum. Dis.* 1982: **8**, 91–103
3. Zein N, Ganuza C and Kushner J. Significance of serum C-reactive protein elevation in patients with SLE. *Arthritis Rheum.* 1979: **22**, 7–12
4. Nived O, Sturfelt G and Wollheim F. Systemic lupus erythematosus and infection: A controlled and prospective study including an epidemiological group. *Q. J. Med.* 1985: **35**, 271–287

1.12   FINGER ON THE PULSE

History

At the age of 7 a girl presented with bruising and thrombocytopaenia. Despite thorough investigation by the paediatricians, a substantive diagnosis was not made. At 16, this recurred along with epistaxis, malaise and tendonitis. Steroids were given but the thrombocytopaenia persisted and she underwent splenectomy a year later. Her condition improved but 4 years later she re-presented with florid SLE, characterized by arthritis, alopecia, migraine, subcutaneous vasculitis and transient cerebral ischaemic episodes. Remission was induced on high-dose oral steroids (40 mg prednisolone daily). This was tailed off, but over the next few years her clinical course was punctuated by disease flares which were always accompanied by profound thrombocytopaenia.

She was referred to the rheumatology unit when on one occasion the thrombocytopaenia persisted despite resolution of other disease features on prednisolone.

Progress and management (Figure 1.12)

Initially she was treated with intravenous methylprednisolone (IVMP), one gram on three consecutive days and over the next week her symptoms gradually improved. Her platelet count rose quickly, reaching a peak of 395 x 10^9/L nine days after the first dose of IVMP. She was discharged and followed up in the clinic on a reducing dose of oral prednisolone (initially 20 mg per day).

Four months later she developed a flare of the disease, her platelet count falling to 9 x 10^9/L. She was treated with a single pulse of IVMP, which was followed by a rise in platelet count to 75 x 10^9/L. Because this rise was not maintained, she was given two further pulses seven and nine days after the first. Her platelet count rose more slowly than previously, peaking at 337 x 10^9/L.

Approximately nine months later, the patient had yet another flare, characterized by tendonitis, arthritis and thrombocytopaenia (15 x 10^9/L). She was given three further pulses of IVMP on consecutive days. Her symptoms improved, but on this occasion the platelet count only rose to 141 x 10^9/L (fourth day after first pulse).

33

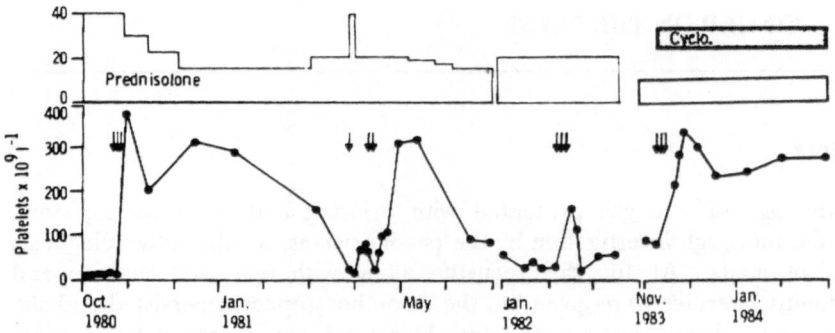

Figure 1.12 Platelet count in response to IVMP, together with concurrent dose of prednisolone. Arrows indicate a single dose (1 mg) of IVMP. 'Cyclo' indicates cyclophosphamide therapy (Reproduced from reference 5 by kind permission of the publishers)

At the end of this period she developed proteinuria, a rising serum creatinine, an active urinary sediment, and mild hypertension. A renal biopsy showed a diffuse proliferative glomerulonephritis with crescent formation. Her platelet count was 88×10^9/L.

She was given a fourth course of IVMP, and started on oral cyclophosphamide at a dose of 2.5 mg kg^{-1} day^{-1}. Her platelet count rose to 346×10^9/L, the creatinine and urinary sediment returned to normal, and the proteinuria diminished.

She continues to be followed up in the clinic. At no time have antiplatelet antibodies been detected. Her most recent platelet count was 288×10^9/L.

Points for discussion

This woman illustrates some challenges and difficulties in the treatment of SLE.

IVMP was first used for the treatment of SLE in the mid-1970s. Initially it was given to patients with lupus nephritis but has subsequently been used in cases with other features of lupus, such a lung disease and cerebral disease. However its successful use has been reported in two patients with SLE whose disease was characterized by a predominant thrombocytopaenia. Fessel *et al.* reported a patient with thrombocytopaenia due to SLE who was treated on three separate occasions with high-dose dexamethasone. The treatment produced an increase in platelets each time, although its efficacy appeared to be dose-related.

34

Our patient is of interest in that she received three separate courses of IVMP specifically for her thrombocytopaenia, as well as a fourth course for a subsequent nephritis. We therefore had the opportunity of observing the effect of repeated courses of IVMP upon SLE-related thrombocytopaenia.

Many authors have stressed the major advantages of IVMP compared with high-dose oral steroids: an increased therapeutic effect accompanied by a relatively low incidence of steroid-associated side-effects. Serious complications of IVMP therapy are probably uncommon; in particular, aseptic necrosis appears to be rare (although time may change this impression).

There have been few reports on the effect of repeated courses of IVMP in SLE. In the patient reported here, the therapy was notably free of complications.

Comment

This case suggests that a degree of tolerance to the drug may develop, resulting in a diminishing response of certain features of the disease to repeated courses of IVMP.

The autoimmune thrombocytopaenia of SLE does not respond to splenectomy as favourably as in ITP. Before embarking on this procedure, it is advisable to explore other avenues of therapy if long-term remission is not maintained on steroid therapy, such as vincristine, vinblastine, danazol or plasmapheresis. This case illustrates the therapeutic dilemma occuring in such a patient and the diminishing response to 'pulse' therapy.

References

1. Cathcart E S, Idelson B A, Scheinberg M A and Couser W G. Beneficial effects of methylprednisolone 'pulse' therapy in diffuse proliferative lupus nephritis. *Lancet* 1976: **1**, 163–166
2. Eyanson S, Passo M H, Aldo-Benson M A and Benson M D. Methylprednisolone pulse therapy for non renal lupus erythematosus. *Ann. Rheum. Dis.* 1980: **39**, 377–380
3. Fessel W J. Megadose corticosteroid therapy in systemic lupus erythematosus. *J. Rheumatol.* 1980: **1**, 486–500
4. Kimberley R P. Pulse methylprednisolone in SLE. *Clin. Rheum. Dis.* 1980: **1**, 390
5. Mackworth Young C G, Walport M J and Hughes G R V. Thrombocytopaenia in a case of systemic lupus erythematosus: Repeated administration of 'pulse' methyl prednisolone. *Br. J. Rheumatol.* 1984: **23**, 298–300
6. Hall S, McCormick J L, Greipp P R, Michet C J and McKenna C H. Splenectomy does not cure the thrombocytopaenia of systemic lupus erythematosus. *Ann. Intern. Med.* 1985: **102**, 325–328

1.13 LUPUS AND LYMPHOMA

History

Mrs A.W., a 39-year-old Asian shopkeeper, presented to her local hospital with exertional dyspnoea and malaise. She was found to have a Hb of 7 g/dl and was transferred with symptomatic improvement. Two months later she was seen again in the clinic. She had lost weight and had intermittent fevers. She complained of aching and stiffness in the small joints of her hands and her knees, and on examination she had a diffuse patchy erythematous rash, and marked cervical and inguinal lymphadenopathy. Once again she was anaemic. She was referred for further evaluation.

On going into the history in more detail, she had been unwell for almost a year. She had always suffered with winter bronchitis, but had developed multiple antibiotic hypersensitivities. In addition to the clinical finding described above, she had a palpable spleen and alopecia of her scalp.

Investigations

Hb	9 g/dl. macrocytosis
WC	normal
Platelets	normal
ESR	95 mm/h
B_{12}	normal
Folate	normal
Coombs' test	positive
Haptoglobulins	absent
Marrow	erythroid hyperplasia
[51]Cr studies	reduced RBC survival
ANA	positive (1:640)

Progress and management

The positive Coombs' test and absent haptoglobulins suggested a haemolytic anaemia. This was supported by a marrow with erythroid hyperplasia and reduced red cell survival on ^{51}Cr studies. When her ANA was found to be strongly positive, a probable diagnosis of SLE was made and she was started on high-dose steroids. Although her Hb improved, she remained unwell and sustained intermittent fevers. A lymph node biopsy was abnormal, and a haematological diagnosis of angioimmunoblastic lymphadenopathy (AILD) was made. She received numerous courses of chemotherapy, but to no avail, and died a year later.

Points for discussion

AILD was first described in 1975 and is an unusual variant of Hodgkin's. It carries a poor prognosis with less than 20% of patients surviving more than 3 years. Clinically patients present, much as in this case, with fever, weight loss, a variety of rashes, generalized lymphadenopathy and hepatosplenomegaly. At least 50% have evidence of a Coombs'-positive haemolytic anaemia, and most have a polyclonal increase in gammaglobulins, presumably accounting for the positive ANA in this patient. In one third, a history of drug hypersensitivity may be elucidated. Diagnosis is made histologically, and, although there may be a transient response to steroids, chemotherapy on the whole is of no benefit.

The incidence of lymphomas arising within the spectrum of connective tissue diseases, such as rheumatoid, SLE and Sjögren's syndrome, is almost certainly increased, although most studies are based on small series or case reports. One major review suggests an increased incidence of 3.7% in SLE compared with 1.36% in controls. The relationship to immunosuppressive treatment is unclear. The occurrence of pseudolymphomas in Sjögren's syndrome is discussed in Case 3.3 and of non-Hodgkins lymphoma in the same syndrome in Cases 3.4 and 3.5.

Comment

My own impression is that lymphoma is surprisingly rare in SLE, considering the immunological and therapeutic challenges facing these patients.

SLE is now one of the world's more common major medical diseases, yet the number of reported complicating lymphomas is small.

Further reading

1. Lukes R J and Collins R D. New approaches to classification of lymphoma. *Cancer* 1975: **31**, Suppl II, 1 – 28
2. Lewis R B, Cator C S, Kinsley R E *et al*. Frequency of neoplasia in SLE and RA. *Arthritis Rheum.* 1979: **19**, 1256 – 1260

3. Rosenstein E D, Wieczornek R, Raphael B and Agus B. Systemic lupus erythematosus and angioimmunoblastic lymphadenopathy: case report and review of the literature. *Semin. Arthritis Rheum.* 1986: **16**, 146–151
4. Frizzera G, Moran E M and Rappaport H. Angioimmunoblastic lymphadenopathy. *Am. J. Med.* 1975: **59**, 803–818

1.14   USE OF ANTIMALARIAL DRUGS

History

A 19-year-old chambermaid was referred to the rheumatology unit from Glasgow as she had moved to London to work. Three years earlier a diagnosis of SLE had been made when she developed a photosensitive rash and arthritis. A year later she was admitted with nephritis and cerebral disease manifesting as status epilepticus. This was treated with a combination of plasma exchange and steroids. A year before coming to London, she had become depressed, developed a further episode of acute glomerulonephritis and a polyneuropathy which responded to further plasma exchanges and 'pulse' cyclophosphamide therapy.

Progress and management

In 1983, when she was first seen in our lupus clinic, she was in remission on only 5 mg prednisolone a day. As this was further reduced, her malar rash returned, she felt tired and had polyarthralgias. There was no proteinuria. Rather than increase her steroids, she was entered into a double-blind study comparing the effects of OH-chloroquine (4 mg kg^{-1} day^{-1}) for 6 months against placebo. This was a carefully supervised study, with monthly clinic attendances and was undertaken by the patient with full informed consent. During the first 6 months, her symptoms improved dramatically and the prednisolone was withdrawn completely. Over this period her DNA binding was stable at 50% (NR<20%) and she had a normal complement profile. Three weeks after changing to the second half of the study, her DNA binding rose to 95% with evidence of complement consumption. Two weeks later she developed an active nephritis with proteinuria of nephrotic proportions. This responded to pulsed IVMP as previously described and an increase in prednisolone to 20 mg daily.

Points for discussion

The use of chloroquine and hydroxychloroquine in the rheumatic diseases was well known in the past although there have been but few adequate controlled studies of its efficacy. In SLE there has been a recent resurgence of interest, in particular in 'mild disease' where skin and synovium are the primary targets.

The way in which these drugs work is unclear but probably multifactorial. Retinal toxicity used to disuade people from its use. Oculotoxicity is due to deposition of the drug in the pigmented tissue of the uveal tract with resultant degeneration of rods and cones. Although retinal damage is extremely rare if the drugs are used in low doses (chloroquine <6 mg kg^{-1} day^{-1}) and OH-chloroquine <4 mg kg^{-1} day^{-1}), six monthly ophthalmic assessment is still recommended. Other side effects include mild gastrointestinal upset, cycloplegia, a neuromyopathy and rarely myasthenia. Its use in pregnancy is controversial.

The use of antimalarials in the more severe spectrum of SLE is also controversial. This particular patient, however, did well, as we found on 'unblinding' the study, and this anecdotally suggests that OH-chloroquine may have been adequately controlling her potentially severe disease. We have since encountered another patient with acute SLE and severe active synovitis, necessitating the almost continual use of 'splints' to minimize the pain, and who within 48 hours of starting OH-chloroquine was able to do her gardening again after more than one year of inactivity.

Comment

Antimalarials have come to be a therapeutic cornerstone in mild to moderate disease.

References

1. Dubois E L. Quinacrine in treatment of systemic and discoid lupus erythematosus. *Arch. Intern. Med.* 1954: **94**, 131
2. Lanham J G and Hughes G R V. Antimalarial therapy in SLE. *Clin. Rheum. Dis.* 1982: **8**, 279–298
3. Conte J J, Mignon-Conte M A and Fournie G J. Lupus nephritis. Treatment with indomethacin-hydroxychloroquine combination, and comparison with corticosteroid treatment. *Nouv. Presse Med.* 1975: **4**, 91
4. Rynes R I. Antimalarial treatment of rheumatoid arthritis 1985 status. *J. Rheumatol.* 1985: **12** (4), 657–658

1.15   CHRONIC CUTANEOUS LE – THE TREATMENT OPTIONS

History

Mrs G.H. presented aged 34 with a history of facial rash at the age of 24 diagnosed as discoid lupus. At this time, there were no serological abnormalities. The diagnosis was made clinically and she was treated with prednisolone. Three years later she developed severe Raynaud's phenomenon particularly affecting the first and second fingers of the left hand. This was sufficiently severe to suggest a proximal arterial lesion and an arch aortogram was performed, which was normal. Serology again proved negative. Aged 29, she underwent bilateral upper dorsal sympathectomy for her Raynaud's, at which time she was found to have an elevated ESR, hyperglobulinaemia and circulating anti-DNA antibodies. A lupus band test showed IgM and complement deposition at the dermoepidermal junction.

Over the year prior to her presentation, her skin rash worsened markedly and proved resistant to both topical and systemic corticosteroids, antimalarials and azathioprine.

Investigations

ESR	100 mm/h
Hb	13.2 g/dl
WC	4.7×10^9/L (lymphocytes 0.5)
ANA	positive 1:80, homogenous pattern
DNA antibody	>94 units/ml
Crithidia DNA	positive (titre >1:160)
Chest X-ray, ECG and renal function	normal

Progress and management

This lady presented the clinical problem of serologically active lupus with organ involvement apparently entirely restricted to the skin. Initially atabrin 50 mg/day was added to her pre-existing treatment of hydroxychloroquine 200 mg once daily. This was ineffective. Subsequently, the steroids were increased with an apparent initial improvement. However, later the rash deteriorated again and she was unable to walk because of severe tenderness and ulceration of her feet. Her serology remained active.

The possibility of a superimposed drug reaction due to the antimalarials was raised. Antimalarials were stopped and dapsone 100 mg/day was instituted. Over the next two weeks, this produced a marked improvement in her rash. However, while still in hospital she developed the sudden onset of central chest pain and was found to have a pericardial rub. Pericarditis resolved with the re-institution of high dose steroids 40 mg/day, which were subsequently tapered. Six weeks later she became anaemic with a reticulocyte count of 30%. This was attributed to the dapsone which was temporarily stopped and then reinstituted at a lower dosage without recurrence of major haemolysis and she was later able to resume the full dosage of 100 mg/day. By this time her ESR had fallen to 30, Hb 10.8, serology remained active, DNA antibody 88 units/ml, crithidia DNA 1:160.

Points for discussion

Cutaneous SLE is frequently responsive to antimalarials with or without topical corticosteroids. Resistant cases pose a difficult therapeutic problem.

We have found the simultaneous use of mepacrine and hydroxy-chloroquine helpful in this situation. Other treatments successfully employed are: clofazimine, thalidomide and most recently dapsone. The latter drug appears effective even in low doses. We obtained a gratifying response with dapsone in what had become a depressing situation for the patient unable to work or walk far because of the discomfort from her rash.

Comment

The response of many patients with chronic cutaneous LE to a variety of drugs mentioned above is often extremely prompt and gratifying.

References

1. Gilliam J N and Sontheimer R D. Distinctive cutaneous subsets in the spectrum of lupus erythematosus. *J. Am. Acad. Dermatol.* 1981: 4, 471–475
2. Crovato F and Levi L. Clofazinine in the treatment of annular lupus erythematosus. *Arch. Dermatol.* 1981: 117, 249
3. Hasper M F. Chronic cutaneous lupus erythematosus – thalidomide treatment of 11 patients. *Arch. Dermatol.* 1983: 119, 812–815
4. Coburn P R and Shuster S. Dapsone and DLE. *Br. J. Dermatol.* 1982: 106, 105–106
5. McCormick L S, Elgart M L and Turner M L C. Annular subacute cutaneous lupus erythematosus responsive to dapsone. *J. Am. Acad. Dermatol.* 1984: 2, 397–401
6. Fenton D A, Shaw M and Black M M. Low dose Dapsone in the treatment of subacute cutaneous lupus erythematosus. *Clin. Exp. Dermatol.* 1985: 10, 279–283

Section 2

SJÖGREN'S SYNDROME

INTRODUCTION

Sjögren's syndrome (SS) results from the destruction of exocrine glands resulting from lymphocyte infiltration. It may occur alone, when it is referred to as 'primary', or in association with other autoimmune disease, when it is 'secondary', particularly with SLE, rheumatoid arthritis, systemic sclerosis and dermato/polymyositis. It is a common accompaniment of chronic biliary cirrhosis and may be associated with thyroiditis, lipodystrophy and graft-versus-host disease. Additionally, 'Sicca-like' symptoms have been noted in a variety of conditions, such as haemochromatosis, sarcoidosis, amyloidosis and type V hyperlipoproteinaemia.

'Sicca' complaints are not uncommon in the elderly, consequent to a decrease in salivary/lacrimal gland function as a normal part of the aging process. It should also be borne in mind that oral dryness may be a common complaint in individuals receiving certain medications and among depressed patients.

Glands affected are predominantly the lacrimal and salivary glands, but other organs involved include the stomach and pancreas, leading to atrophic gastritis and pancreatitis. Abnormality of secretions of the upper and lower respiratory tract may lead to dryness of the nose, throat and trachea. Otitis, bronchitis, pneumonitis and recurrent vaginitis may occur. Epistaxis and nasal 'crusting' may be symptomatic of nasal dryness. Pulmonary involvement with multiple infiltrates or fibrosis can occur; other organs may be involved in the so-called 'extraglandular' syndrome.

The kidney may be affected with interstitial lymphocytic infiltrates leading to an interstitial nephritis, tubular atrophy and fibrosis, presenting with hyposthenuria, renal tubular acidosis, a Fanconi syndrome and, rarely, there may be defective renal function resulting from membranous or membrano-proliferative glomerulonephritis.

Hepatic involvement with round cell portal infiltration and fibrosis has been documented (with raised Alk.PO_4).

A myopathic syndrome, usually unaccompanied by elevation of muscle enzymes, has been described and peripheral neuropathy, which is usually mild, symmetrical and predominantly sensory, with a particular predilection for the trigeminal nerve (when it may be bilateral) has also been documented.

Of great interest recently has been the recognition of the frequency of vasculitis in patients with 'primary' Sjögren's syndrome and mononeuritis multiplex, purpura, gangrene and glomerulonephritis may be manifestations of this complication. There is often cryoglobulinaemia. Thyroid abnormalities with consequent hypothyroidism have been documented in 10–15% of patients and it is thought that lymphoid infiltrates producing Hashimoto's thyroiditis is the underlying aetiology. Antibodies to thyroglobulin a thyroid microsomes may be present and thyroid-stimulating hormone (TSH) levels may be elevated in a large proportion of patients.

Manifestations of B-cell hyperactivity are common and include polyclonal hypergammaglobulinaemia, the production of non-specific organ auto-antibodies, such as rheumatoid factor and antinuclear antibodies (ANA) and the presence of antibodies to extractable nuclear antigens (ENAs), particularly to Ro (SS-A) and La (SS-B), as well as elevated salivary IgA.

The prevalence of antibodies to the ENAs Ro and La in patients with primary and secondary Sjögren's has varied in different studies, but recently Whittingham *et al.* found a strong correlation between the presence of the La antibody and primary Sjögren's. It did not occur in patients with RA or with primary biliary cirrhosis and was found infrequently in association with other autoimmune diseases. It was strongly linked to the phenotype HLA-B8, DR3. Antibodies to Ro appeared to correlate strongly with a high prevalence of extraglandular disease and vasculitis.

Diagnosis of the condition is by Schirmer's test and by salivolabial biopsy in which typical lymphocytic infiltration may be seen. Sequential salivary scintigraphy is also useful. This is measured one hour after the i.v. injection of ^{99}Tc partechnetate. This procedure correlates well with labial salivary gland pathology and reduction of parotid flow rates may be seen spont-aneously or following stimulation with acid drops.

A variety of malignant lymphomas and other tumours have complicated Sjögren's syndrome and the risk appears to be 6.4 cases per 100 per year. These may be of varying histological types. Waldenström's macroglobulin-aemia has been described as well as a 'pseudolymphoma' where the cells have also been shown to be of B-cell origin. In pseudolymphoma and angio-blastic lymphadenopathy, there appears to be a high frequency of progression to frank lymphoma.

Further reading

1. Moutsopoulos H M, Chused T M, Mann D L et al. Sjögren's syndrome (sicca syndrome): Current issues. *Ann. Intern. Med.* 1980: 92, 212–226
2. Alexander E, Arnett F, Provost T and Stevens M B. Sjögren's syndrome: association with anti-Ro (SS-A) antibodies with vasculitis, haematological abnormalities and serologic hyperreactivity. *Ann. Intern. Med.* 1983: 98, 155–159
3. Fox R I, Howell F V, Bone R C et al. Primary Sjögren's syndrome: clinical and immunolopathologic features. *Semin. Arthritis Rheum.* 1984: 14, 77–105
4. Fox R I, Robinson C A and Curd J G. Sjögren's syndrome. Proposed criteria for classification. *Arthritis Rheum.* 1986: 29, 577–585

2.1 FACIAL NUMBNESS

History

At 35 years, this woman presented to her GP with increasing numbness over her face and scalp. Initially this was patchy, but it progressively became more widespread. Ten years earlier she had developed similar symptoms in the right foot and left hand. There was a past history of mild Raynaud's phenomenon, but she had not noticed any grittiness of her eyes or excessive dryness of the mouth or thirst. There had been no joint symptoms.

Clinical abnormalities were confined to the nervous system. Both pupils were irregular and reacted poorly to light and both corneal reflexes were absent. Sensation to pain and touch were absent bilaterally in the trigeminal distribution, but there was no facial weakness. Peripherally, there was no wasting, and tone, power and co-ordination were normal. All tendon reflexes, however, were absent. Appreciation of pain and touch were lost in a glove and stocking distribution. Vibration sense was absent below the knees and proprioception absent in toes, ankles, fingers and wrists. Romberg's test was positive.

Investigations

Hb	12.2 g/dl
WC	4.2×10^9/L
ESR	19 mm/h
Immunoglobulins	elevated with IgM 5.6 g/dl
Latex test	positive (1:320)
ANA	positive (1:320)
DNA binding	15%
ENA	positive (for anti-Ro)
VDRL	negative
B_{12}/folate levels	normal

Progress and management

CSF studies were normal, as were a CT brain scan and visually evoked responses. An EMG was consistent with peripheral neuropathy. In view of the abnormal serology, a Schirmer's test was performed. This was dry and a biopsy of a buccal salivary gland showed lymphocytic infiltration consistent with a diagnosis of Sjögren's syndrome. X-rays of hands and feet were normal.

She was started on prednisolone, and at follow-up 2 years later there had been no progression of her neurological symptoms.

Points for discussion

Many of the connective tissue diseases are complicated by neurological involvement, and this is also documented in Sjögren's syndrome (SS), occuring in up to a quarter of patients. The best description of the neurological features is by Kaltreider and Talal who described peripheral neuropathy in 10 out of 1098 patients with SS. It was usually symmetrical and predominantly sensory. In 5 patients there was involvement of the cranial nerves, and the trigeminal nerve was affected in all but one of these. Other series also highlight this predilection of the fifth cranial nerve. Interestingly, this patient did not have symptomatic xerophthalmia, despite lachrymal involvement.

Comment

Facial pain of trigeminal distribution is not uncommon in SLE, MCTD and Sjögren's syndrome. Although some patients respond to steroids, as in this patient, this is not always the case.

References

1. Kaltreider H B and Talal N. The neuropathy of Sjögren's syndrome. Trigeminal nerve involvement. *Ann. Intern. Med.* 1969: **70**, 751–762
2. Alexander W L, Provost T T, Stevens M B and Alexander G E. Neurological complications of primary Sjögren's syndrome. *Medicine (Baltimore)* 1982: **61**, 247–257
3. Ashworth B and Tait G B W. Trigeminal neuropathy in connective tissue diseases. *Neurology* 1971: **21**, 609–614

2.2   LUPUS OR NOT?

History

A 56-year-old Sikh was first seen in the rheumatology department 10 years ago when she had malaise, weight loss, arthralgias and Raynaud's phenomenon. She was anaemic, had a positive latex test for rheumatoid factor and low-titre ANA. A diagnosis of SLE was made on the basis of these findings. A moderately elevated DNA binding (46%) was found on one occasion only and this was during the first week of using this test in our laboratory. Because of hypertension, proteinuria and a low creatinine, a renal biopsy was preformed. This revealed focal glomerulonephritis. She was treated with prednisolone. The hypertension was controlled with a variety of antihypertensive medications.

In 1979 the steroids were stopped, and she remained well until 1981 when she developed fevers and weight loss. She had hepatosplenomegaly and lymphadenopathy.

Investigations

Hb	10.8 g/dl
ESR	118 mm/h
ANA	positive 1:640 (speckled pattern)
Latex test	positive
ENAs	positive for Ro, La
Immunoglobulins	IgG 26 g/dl with IgA 2.9 g/L
Schirmer's test	dry
Salivary gland biopsy	lymphocytic infiltrates

Repeat DNA binding tests and DNA antibodies were consistently negative, and a revised diagnosis of primary Sjögren's syndrome was entertained. Steroids were reintroduced with clinical improvement.

In 1982, her dose of prednisolone had been reduced to 6 mg daily. She was admitted as an emergency with a two week history of epistaxis, bruising and finally a haematemesis. The platelet count on admission was $7 \times 10^9/L$. A sternal marrow showed increased megakaryocyte activity, and anti-platelet antibodies were detected. The prednisolone was increased to 60 mg daily.

Progress and management

Her platelet count rose to acceptable levels, but fell as soon as attempts to withdraw the steroids were made. She became increasingly cushingoid and hypertensive, and a splenectomy was performed. This allowed some reduction in maintenance dose of steroids. Azathioprine was added and the combination resulted in a stable platelet count ranging from 100 to 120 x 10^9/L.

Points for discussion

This woman had many features typical of primary Sjögren's syndrome, including multiple serological abnormalities with antinuclear antibodies, rheumatoid factors, anti-Ro and anti-La antibodies. Low titres of antibody to double-stranded DNA have been documented in this condition and may explain the single elevation of antibodies to ds DNA found, if indeed this was not a laboratory error.

Thrombocytopaenia is well documented in association with SLE but rarely complicates primary Sjögren's. Splenectomy may be of value in some patients, but in this case failed to induce a remission sufficient to allow a drastic reduction in the steroid dose.

Bruising and purpura may occur in Sjögren's syndrome when there is profound hypergammaglobulinaemia despite a normal platelet count – 'purpura hypergammaglobulinaemia '.

Renal involvement is common in Sjögren's syndrome. Apart from renal tubular acidosis, whichg may be overt or incomplete and can be correlated with hypergammaglobulinaemia, sporadic cases of immune complex nephritis have been reported in the absence of any evidence of SLE. The lesions may be membranous or focal proliferative as in our patient.

Comment

This patient has a connective tissue disease with the production of a number of autoantibodies and 'overlap' features. It may be considered academic to attempt precise pigeon-holing of such cases. However, these patients are prone to occasional life-threatening features.

Splenectomy for the thrombocytopaenia of such patients is still unpredictable in its medium- to long-term benefit.

References

1. Nichols C and Brightman V J. Parotid calcifications and cementomas in a patient with Sjögren's syndrome and idiopathic thrombocytopaenic purpura. *J. Oral Pathol.* 1977: **6**, 51-60
2. Moutsopoulos H, Balow J E, Lawley T J *et al.* Immune complex glomerulonephritis in Sicca syndrome. *Am. J. Med.* 1978: **64**, 955-960
3. Bailey R R. Renal involvement in Sjögren's syndrome. *NZ J. Med.* 1986: **99**, 579-580

2.3   A SURPRISING CHOLECYSTECTOMY

History

In 1935, Mrs D.L. developed a sudden illness with arthralgias, lymphadenopathy, a pleural effusion, cutaneous vasculitis and depression. SLE was
diagnosed and prednisolone started. She had recurrent disease flares,
characterized by pleurisy, fevers, leucopaenia and lymphadenopathy. DNA
binding never exceeded 30% (NR < 20%).

In 1979, she was admitted for investigation of proteinuria (2 g/24 h). A
renal biopsy demonstrated a focal glomerulonephritis. Four years later she
developed nausea and upper abdominal pain, as well as severe perimeno-
pausal symptoms. There were no joint deformities, but she had 5 cm
splenomegaly and was tender in the right upper quadrant. She had a mild
anaemia and high-titre ANA at 1:10 000, although tests for antibodies to
ENAs were negative. The Schirmer's test was dry, and biopsy of a minor
salivary gland was consistent with Sjögren's syndrome. Ultrasound
examination of the gall bladder confirmed the clinical impression of gall
stones.

Progress and management

The gall stones were removed at laparotomy, but she had extensive
intra-abdominal lymphadenopathy with a mass of nodes at the porta hepatis.
The surgeon, in fact, thought that these were lymphomatous and several
biopsies were taken. Normal lymph node architecture was preserved but
there was marked immunoblastic proliferation consistent with a diagnosis of
'pseudolymphoma'. One year later the patient developed cervical adenopathy
which showed typical lymphoma on biopsy. She was treated with
chemotherapy and remains well two years later.

Points for discussion

This patient's illness presented with SLE. Several years after the development
of glomerulonephritis, symptoms of SS predominated more than 40 years
after her original presentation.

Lymph node involvement may be a prominent feature of Sjögren's

51

syndrome. In most patients, lymphoproliferation is confined to the salivary and lachrymal glands, but this may extend to affect nodes and other organs if the disease course is extended, and, on occasions, differentiation from a lymphoma may be extremely difficult, and may result in the need for local irradiation or immunosuppressive treatment. Occasionally pseudolymphoma may progress to a malignant lesion, usually accompanied by a fall in titres of rheumatoid factor and IgM.

Comment

Earlier series highlighted lymphoma development as an important feature of Sjögren's syndrome. Our own feeling is that this complication is fortunately rare, but early diagnosis and treatment is important if a fatal outcome is to be avoided.

References

1. Anderson L G and Talal N. The spectrum of benign to malignant lymphoproliferation in Sjögren's syndrome. *Clin. Exp. Immunol.* 1972: 10, 199–221
2. Zulman J, Jaffe R and Talal N. Evidence that the malignant lymphoma of Sjögren's syndrome is a monoclonal B-cell neoplasm. *N. Engl. J. Med.* 1978: 299, 1215–1220
3. Whaley K, Williamson J, Chisholm D M, Webb J, Mason D K, Watson Buchanan W. (1973). Sjögren's syndrome. *Q. J. Med.* 1973: 42, 279–304
4. Whaley K, Webb J, McAvoy B A, Hughes G R V, Lee P, MacSween R N M and Buchanan W W. Sjögren's syndrome. *Q. J. Med.* 1973: 42 (167), 513–548

2.4 SJÖGREN'S AND LYMPHOMA

History

M.M., a 36-year-old Maltese housewife, first presented to hospital with a two-year history of Raynaud's syndrome, seventeen months of dry eyes, and ten months of dry mouth. In the preceding six weeks, the tips of all her fingers had become increasingly ischaemic with evidence of dry gangrene. The only other abnormal clinical sign was widespread minor lymphadenopathy. A diagnosis of Sjögren's syndrome was made. Treatment by prostacycline infusions and bilateral cervical sympathectomies failed to save some fingertips which required amputation. Nifedipine slow-release was started.

Eighteen months later, she was noted to have increased lymphadenopathy and complained of intermittent bilateral parotid gland swelling. Axillary lymph node biopsy showed chronic inflammation only. Some months later, she presented with persistent parotid gland swelling, more widespread lymphadenopathy, fever, weakness, malaise, weight loss and bilateral breast lumps.

Examination revealed a very thin, unwell lady with bilateral parotid swelling (Figure 2.4A); right partial ptosis, large left supraclavicular, axillary, and bilateral inguinal lymphadenopathy; amputated fingertips; left anterior chest wall skin lesions (Figure 2.4A); a mobile mass occupying the whole of the left breast and a small mobile mass in the right breast. There was an enlarged, firm, non-tender liver, and marked generalized wasting and weakness, especially of the legs.

Investigations

WC	normal
ESR	10 mm/h
C-reactive protein	84 mg/L
Alkaline phosphatase	70 IU/L
Alanine transaminase	73 IU/L
Aspartate transaminase	127 IU/L
Albumin	24 g/L
Globulins	18 g/L
IgG	3.5 g/L

53

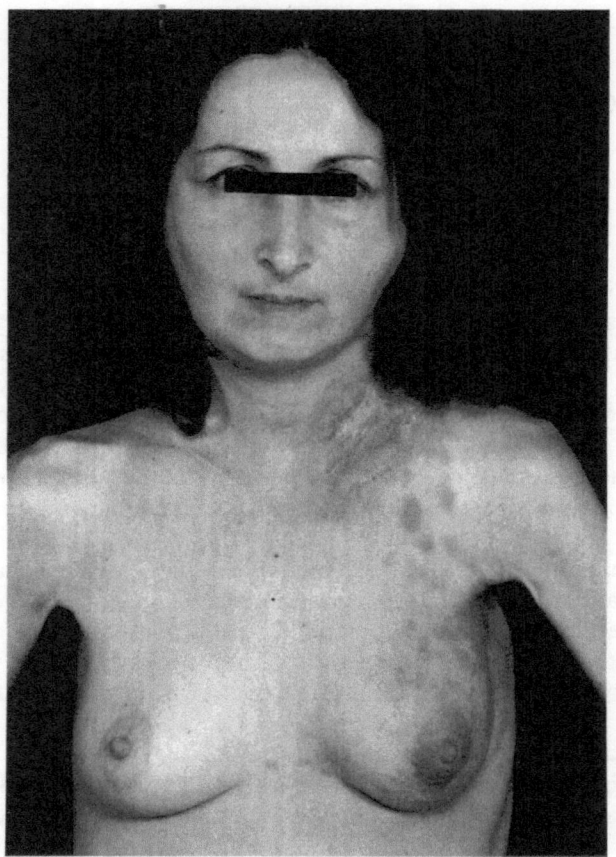

Figure 2.4A Patient showing enlarged parotids

Immunology: ANA	positive (IgG: 1:160 diffuse, IgM: 1:40: speckled and diffuse)
RA latex test:	positive
DNA binding	negative
Complement	normal
Liver ultrasound	liver enlarged with multiple ill-defined hyperechoic areas. Mild splenomegaly, and small amounts of intraperitoneal, pleural and pericardial fluid
Biopsies of skin (Figure 2.4B) and inguinal lymph node (Figure 2.4C)	lymphoid cell infiltration with focal necrosis and vascular proliferation
Immunocytochemistry (Figure 2.4D)	cells positive for cytoplasmic IgM (lambda light chains) and surface IgM

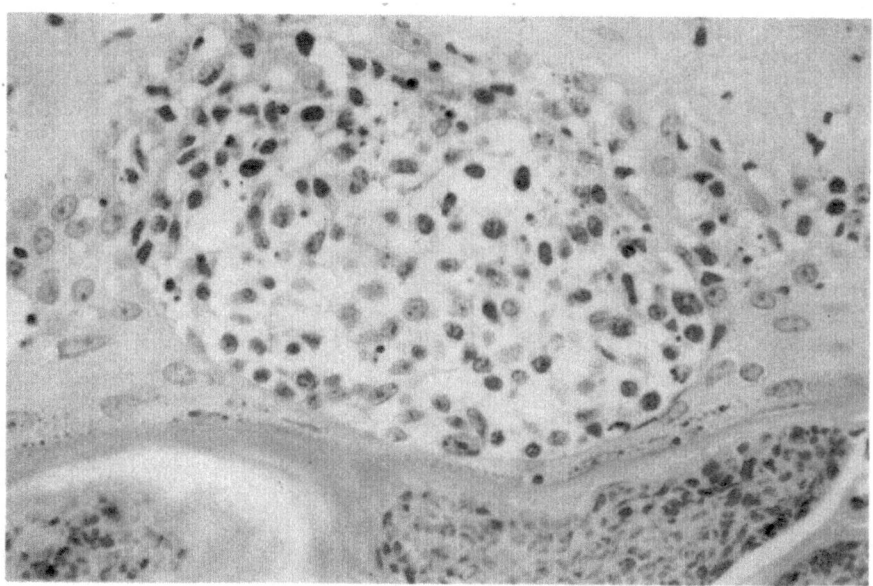

Figure 2.4B Skin biopsy (see text)

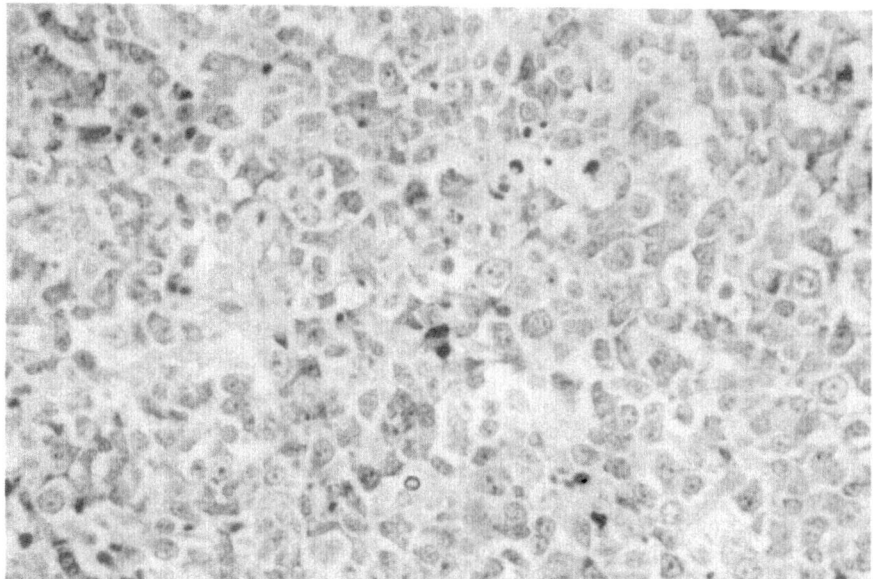

Figure 2.4C Inguinal lymph node biopsy (see text)

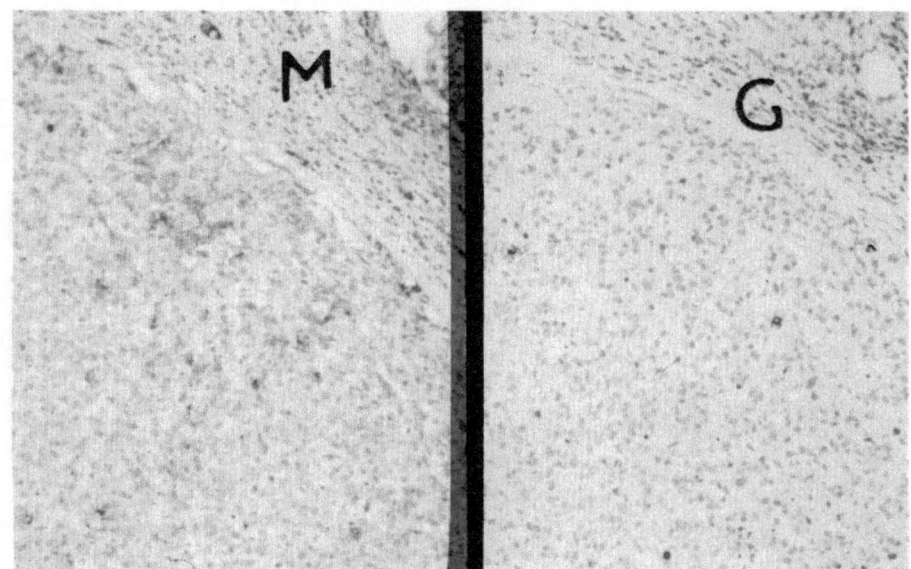

Figure 2.4D Immunocytochemistry: IgM-positive staining cells

Diagnosis

B-cell non-Hodgkin's lymphoma, of a polymorphic centroblastic subtype.

Course

Already extremely weak and unwell at the final presentation, the patient died before chemotherapeutic treatment could be administered for her lymphoma.

Comment

This lady demonstrates one of the rare, but well-recognized complications of Sjögren's syndrome, i.e. malignant lymphomatous change, which may occur in salivary glands or extraglandular tissue. Recurrent parotid swelling and early widespread lymphadenopathy are said to be associated with a higher risk of lymphoma. The latter took a very aggressive course, once established, and was of B-cell origin with lambda light chains, rather than kappa as previously reported. This is distinct from the so-called 'pseudolymphoma'. as documented in the previous case, which lacks the histological criteria of malignant lymphoma, but may mimic it clinically and may respond to steroid therapy. The low immunoglobulins are also characteristic of lymphomatous change in Sjögren's, particularly when levels are high earlier on in the disease.

NB References to this case are included following Case 2.5.

2.5   AN 'AUTOIMMUNE' JOURNEY

C.F., a Caucasian female, first complained of polyarthralgias affecting the hands, knees and ankles at the age of 33 years, followed some 9 years later by the development of bilateral basal reticular shadowing radiologically, a positive antinuclear factor (1:40) and elevated levels of both IgG and IgM proteins. A presumptive diagnosis of fibrosing alveolitis was made. A year later dry 'gritty' eyes and recurrent attacks of conjunctivitis became permanent complaints. A positive Schirmer's test and minor salivary gland biopsy confirmed this diagnosis 5 years later. Features of SLE ('butterfly rash', Raynaud's antibodies to dsDNA, positive Coomb's test) resulted in long-term therapy with prednisolone and azathioprine. Repeated chronic upper respiratory tract infections necessitating frequent hospital admissions were accompanied by multiple drug allergies (penicillin, sulphonamides, tetracyclines). She was referred to St. Thomas' Hospital in 1986, with a resistant infection following catheterization, and repeated anterior nasal crusting and infections.

Examination revealed bilateral basal crepitations, synovitis of small joints of the hands and signs of hypercortisonism ('moon face', buffalo hump, proximal muscle weakness). There was no peripheral adenopathy or salivary gland swelling.

Investigations

Hb	normal
WC	normal
Platelets	normal
ESR	60 mm/h
ANA	negative
DNA binding	negative
ENAs	negative
IgM	elevated, 4.8 g/L
X-rays (Figures 2.5A and B)	Persistent reticular shadowing at bases. Patchy ill-defined shadowing throughout both lung fields
Open lung biopsy	Monomorphic infiltration by sheets of lymphoid cells (Figures 2.5C and D)
Immunocytochemistry	Intracellular IgM demonstrated; cells stain monotypically for Kappa light chains

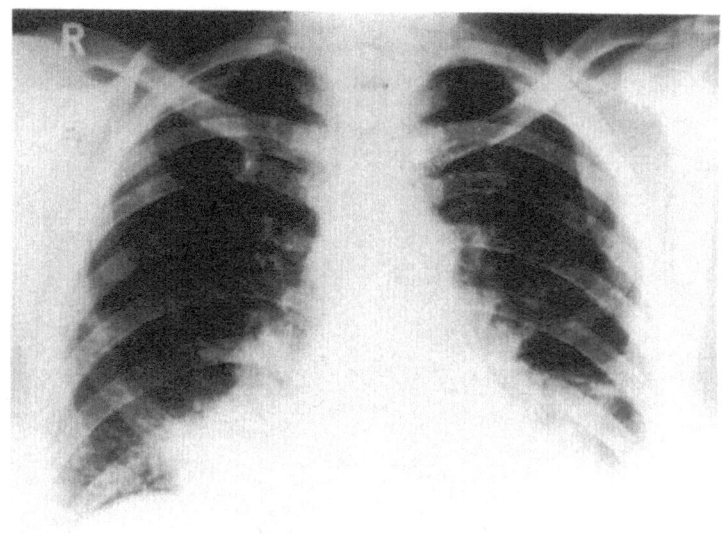

Figure 2.5A Reticular shadowing at both bases, right middle lobe consolidation

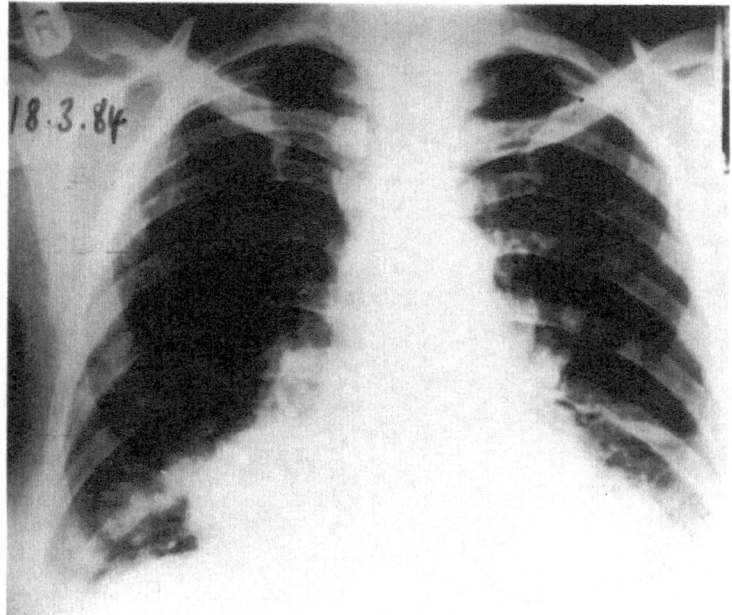

Figure 2.5B Follow-up (2 years later). Small opacities in both lower zones, basal reticular shadowing persists

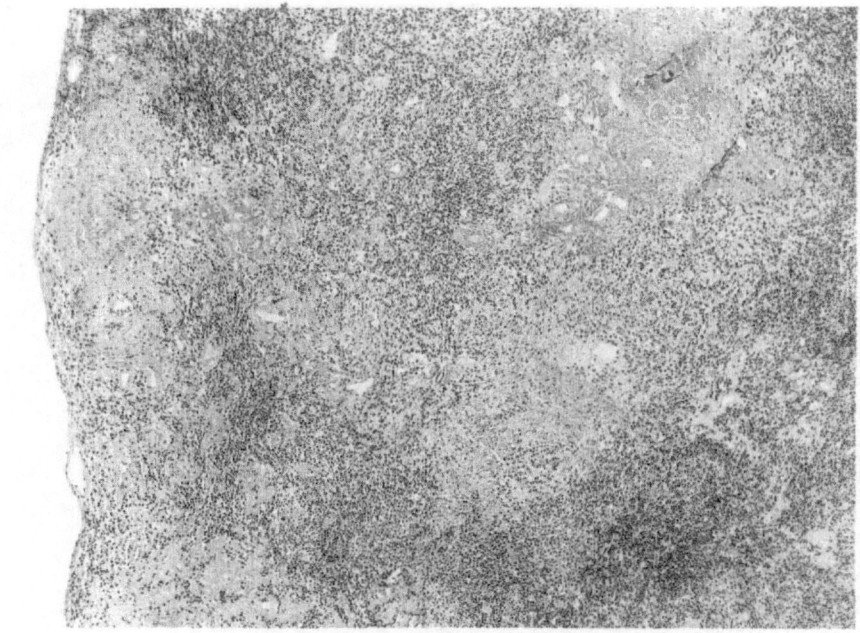

Figure 2.5C Lung and pleura showing destruction of alveolar structure and diffuse replacement by lymphoid cells; note absence of lymphoid follicles

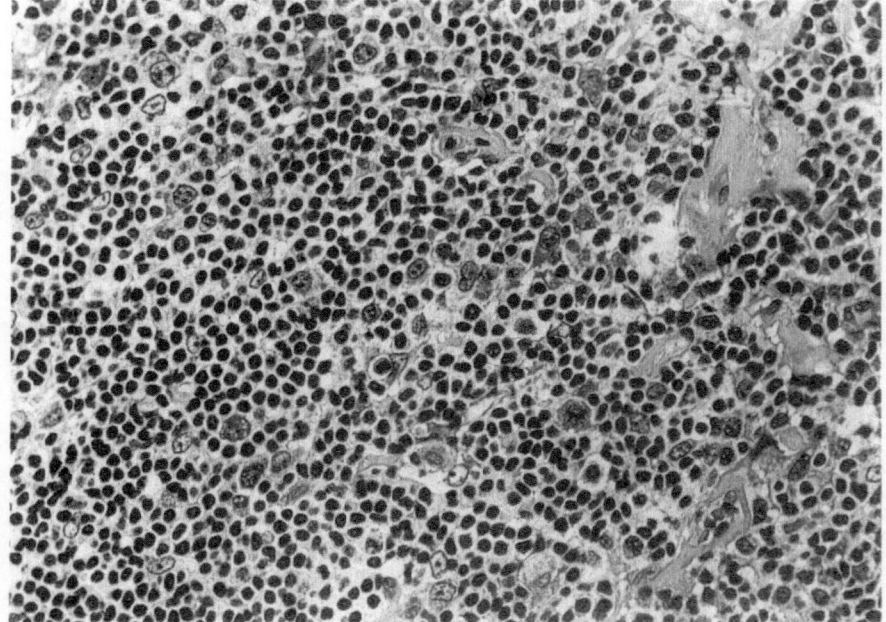

Figure 2.5D Lung. Diffuse replacement by primitive lymphoid cells with large vesicular nuclei and prominent nucleoli x 400

60

Diagnosis

B-cell lymphoma.

Progress and management

The patient was commenced on chlorambucil therapy for the lymphoma but after 9 months of this therapy an increase in pulmonary shadowing was noted (Figure 2.5B). Therapy was altered to cyclophosphamide. Recurrent attacks of respiratory infections again necessitated hospital admissions and the appropriate antibiotic therapy. The patient complained of a painful bridge of the nose, and initial redness and swelling of the nasal cartilage was followed 6 months later by collapse of the nasal bridge.

At no stage were the DNA binding, antibodies to ENAs or ANAs positive.

Points for discussion

This patient's illness demonstrated an unusual combination of 'autoimmune' connective tissue disease over a 20-year period:

Fibrosing alveolitis
Sicca syndrome
Systemic lupus erythematosus
Chondritis,

complicated by the development of B-cell lymphoma of the lung in the absence of salivary gland or superficial lymph gland involvement by the lymphoproliferative process. Additionally, she had been on azathioprine for a number of years. This immunosuppressive has been incriminated in the development of lymphoma, particularly in patients with immunodeficiency, although definitive statistical evidence of this association is still lacking.

First reported by Talal and Bunim in 1964, over 100 cases of the association of a variety of lymphoid abnormalities with Sjögren's syndrome have now been reported, varying from pseudolymphoma to overtly malignant lymphoma, now termed 'immunoblastic immunosarcoma'. Additionally, elevations of the IgM globulins, as was seen in our patient, may be significantly high and be associated with a clinical picture of Waldenström's macroglobulinaemia on occasions.

Recurrent parotid swelling, lymphadenopathy and splenomegaly appear to confer a high risk for the subsequent development of malignancy and a drop in levels of rheumatoid facor and IgM levels may presage the appearance of this malignancy.

The lungs, kidney or gastrointestinal tract may be involved or the salivary glands themselves may be solely affected. In 10% of patients, this may be bilateral and therefore this type of parotid swelling should no longer be regarded as essentially benign. The term myopithelial sialadenitis is now used to describe the histological picture of changes which are seen histologically in the salivary glands. Talal has compared the immunodeficiency seen in the Sicca syndrome with that occurring in the AIDS-related complex (ARC) and the eventual development of the acquired immunodeficiency syndrome (AIDS) polyclonal B-cell activation, immune complexes, increased beta-2-microglobulin, acid-labile interferon, decreased autologous mixed lymphocyte response, decreased interleukin-2 and decreased natural killer cells are similar abnormalities seen in both conditions.

The development of non-Hodgkin's lymphoma has also been documented in patients with SLE, often many years after the initial diagnosis has been made.

Comment

This patient was unusual, not only in the combination of 'autoimmune' disorders manifested clinically, but also in the almost complete lack of polyclonal B-cell stimulation serologically. Thus hypergammaglobulinaemia and positive latex test for rheumatoid factors were always absent and the patient additionally did not demonstrate antibodies to the extractable nuclear antigens Ro and La, so often found in patients with the Sicca syndrome. Chondritis, resulting in the collapse of the nasal bridge, was an interesting clinical development. There was no evidence of polychondritis or granulomatous vasculitis such as Wegener's, and it must, therefore, be attributed to the underlying CT disease.

References

1. Kassan S S, Thomas T L, Moutsopoulos H H, *et al*. Increased risk of lymphoma in Sicca syndrome. *Ann. Intern. Med.* 1978: 39, 888–892
2. Rieche K. Carcinogenicity of antineoplastic agents in man. *Cancer Treatment Rev.* 1984: 11, 39–67
3. Kinlen L J, Skell A G R, Peto R J and Doll R. Collaborative United Kingdom–Australasian study of cancer in patients treated with immunosuppressive drugs. *Br. Med. J.* 1979: 2, 1461–1469

4. Talal N, Sokoloff L and Barton W F. Extrasalivary lymphoid abnormalities in Sjögren's syndrome (reticulum-cell sarcoma, 'pseudolymphoma', macroglobulinaemia). *Am. J. Med.* 1967: **43**, 50 – 65

5. Talal N. The biological significance of lymphoproliferation in Sjögren's syndrome. In P M Brooks and J R York (eds.) *Rheumatology – 85*, pp. 365 – 369. (Elsevier Science Publishers)

6. Green J A, Dawson A A and Walker W. Systemic lupus erythematosus and lymphoma. *Lancet* 1978: 753 – 755

7. Law, N W, Leader M. Bilateral submandibular gland lymphoma in Sjögren's syndrome. *Postgrad. Med. J.* 1987: **63**, 135 – 136

2.6   THE LADY WITH THE LARGE PAROTIDS

History

This 34-year-old lady initially presented to her general practitioner with lymphadenopathy at the age of 21. A presumptive diagnosis of glandular fever was made and she made a slow recovery over 4 months, though over this period she developed myalgia and lost 1 stone in weight. She next presented aged 25 with progressive enlargement of the left parotid gland followed by enlargement of the right, which was also associated with the development of dry eyes and a dry mouth. At the age of 32 she was seen with an acute polyarthritis affecting her hands, knees and feet. This settled over several weeks on non-steroidal anti-inflammatory drugs. The following year she had a further episode of polyarthritis associated with a purpuric rash on the lower legs. Her main complaint, however, was of marked symmetrical parotid enlargement over the two years prior to her presentation to us. The results of her investigations on that visit are listed below.

Investigations

Hb	12.0 g/dl
Platelets	normal (189×10^9/L)
WCC	6.4×10^9/L
ESR	69 mm/h
ANF	negative (1:10)
ENA	positive (Ro and La +ve)
RA latex test	positive (1:256)
Total proteins	normal
Crithidia DNA	negative
Immune complexes (PEG)	26.6 mg IgG/dl
Cryoglobulins	positive
X-rays (chest, wrists, hands)	normal
Schirmer's test	positive (dry)

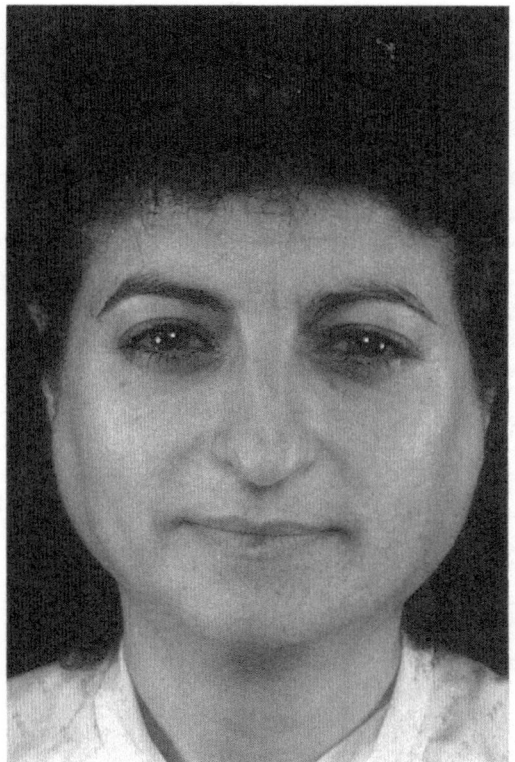

Figure 2.6A Bilateral parotid enlargement

Progress and management

Although the patient had marked parotid enlargement she was otherwise well. No treatment was started on her first visit. She remained well until March 1987 when she presented with a symmetrical polyarthritis affecting her wrists, ankles and neck. She was commenced on prednisolone 15 mg daily and hydroxychloroquine 200 mg and review was arranged for 2 weeks. At that time it was found that not only had her arthritis completely gone but also her face had resumed a normal contour!

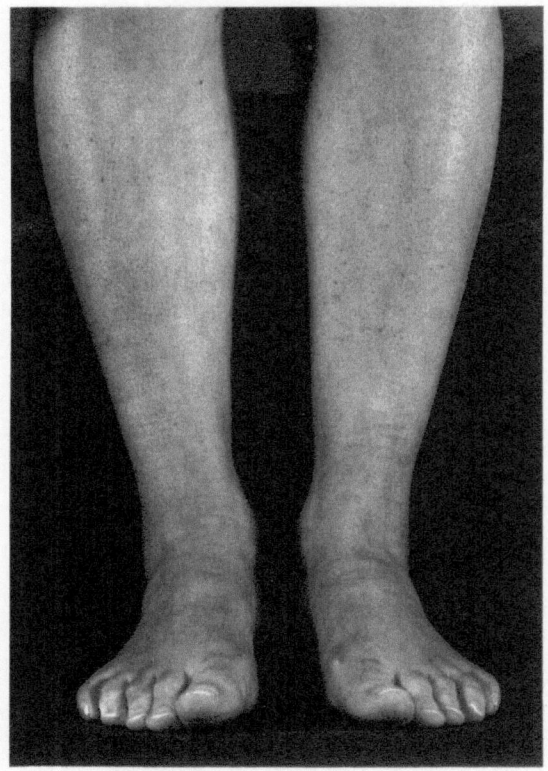

Figure 2.6B Polyarthritis affecting ankles

Comment

Although a dramatic response of parotid enlargement is reported, this is not a consistent finding in Sjögren's syndrome. In view of the otherwise limited therapeutic options, a short course of low-dose steroids is worth a trial.

Reference

1. Kelley E, Harris E D, Ruddy S and Sledge C B (eds.) Sjögren's syndrome. In *Textbook of Rheumatology* 2nd Edn, 1985, Philadelphia, W B Saunders, pp. 971–999

Section 3

RHEUMATOID DISEASE

INTRODUCTION

It has been suggested that RA is becoming less common and possibly less severe – nonetheless it currently affects between 1 and 2% of the adult population.

The clinical challenges of rheumatoid disease occur at several levels. Diagnostically we still rely heavily on rheumatoid factor positivity and the recognition of joint erosions to confirm our clinical suspicions; in the absence of these features, the differential diagnostic net of 'seronegative RA' is wide, from an atypical spondylarthropathy to the occasional presentation of primarily non-rheumatic disorders such as occult malignancy or inflammatory bowel disease.

Prognostically too, clear markers of value in an individual patient are few and far between, particularly in those who primarily have joint disease. For those with clinically apparent 'systemic' features, the picture is somewhat clearer and justifies modern trends towards aggressive drug therapy.

Therapeutically, too, there are real difficulties. We have a number of reasonably effective anti-inflammatory drugs – non-steroid, steroid and so-called second-line – and our understanding of them has encouraged us to use them all more freely in dosages proven by clinical trial to be compatible with reasonable safety and efficacy. But we still do not know if they really influence the outcome of the disease – the most recent long-term follow up suggests that they do *not* to any large extent. This suggests that any future therapy has to influence both the inflammatory and destructive aspects of the rheumatoid process. Cellular immunology and biochemistry are giving us clues as to the nature of the messages immune/inflammatory cells use to activate destructive processes and we will hopefully, therefore, see a whole new class of therapeutic agents in the future.

Meanwhile, we hope that these clinical cases will illustrate the current therapeutic alternatives for RA and the differential diagnostic problems which systemic rheumatoid disease presents to the clinician.

Further reading

1. Scott D L, Symmons D P M, Coulton B L and Popert A J. Long-term outcome of treating rheumatoid arthritis: results after 20 years. *Lancet* 1987: 1, 1108–1111

3.1 APPROACHES TO RHEUMATOID VASCULITIS

History

The patient, a 57-year-old female, had a seven-year history of seropositive nodular rheumatoid arthritis, treated for the first five years with NSAIDs. Because of worsening disease she was started on low-dose systemic corticosteroid therapy followed by one year of D-penicillamine, discontinued because of proteinuria. Thereafter she developed progressive weight loss, increasing joint pains and weakness and paraesthesiae of both arms and legs. A maculopapular rash followed, involving particularly the area of the ankles and feet. Azathioprine was introduced and the steroids increased. Despite this, she deteriorated and was admitted to hospital for treatment.

On clinical examination, she had wasting of the small muscles of the hands with weakness, as well as distal weakness of the legs with absent tendon reflexes. A 'glove and stocking' complete sensory loss was present to the midshins and wrists. The rash over both lower limbs was beginning to ulcerate.

Investigations

Hb	11.5 g/dl. normochromic normocytic
WC	14.4 x 10^9/L (87% neutrophils)
Platelets	570x10^9/L
ESR	72 mm/h
RA latex test	positive (1:320)
ANA	positive (1:520)
DNA	negative
ENAs	negative
Immune complexes	strongly positive for CIq binding
Cryoglobulins	positive
Schirmer's test	dry bilaterally
Buccal gland biopsy	lymphocytic infiltration

Skin biopsy (ulcer, right leg): necrosis of the epidermis and dermis with accompanying thrombosis of vessels.

Progress and management

Treatment with high dose steroids (prednisolone 60 mg/day) and cyclo-phosphamide (2.5 mg kg^{-1} day^{-1}) was started and she was given three 4 L plasma exchanges over three days. This was combined with intensive local and systemic treatment with appropriate antibiotics for superadded infection of the ulcers. There was gradual healing of her ulcers and no progression of the neuropathy. Some power returned to the legs. Her ESR dropped to 25 mm/h and levels of immune complexes fell. Neuralgic pains in her hands and feet became a problem but did not respond to carbamazepine or phenytoin. Over the next three years she was maintained on a small dose of prednisolone although she had residual weakness and sensory loss. Her latex test remained positive (1:160) but immune complexes and cryoglobulins disappeared.

Points for discussion

Systemic vasculitis complicating rheumatoid arthritis is serious and carries an appreciable morbidity and mortality justifying aggressive therapy. The patient illustrates such disease and demonstrates many characteristic features (Table 3.1). Fortunately the full-blown picture is rare.

Table 3.1 Clinical and laboratory features of rheumatoid vasculitis

Weight loss
Cutaneous ulcers
Rheumatoid nodules
Hepatosplenomegaly
Lymphadenopathy
Pericarditis
Visceral and digital infarcts
Neuropathy
Episcleritis and sicca syndrome

Anaemia
Neutrophilia
Thrombocytosis
ESR >100 mm/h
High titre rheumatoid factor
Positive ANA
Circulating immune complexes
Cryoglobulinaemia

Although rheumatoid vasculitis is usually associated with longstanding erosive disease, it may be the initial manifestation of rheumatoid, and carries a poor prognosis.

Controversies in management abound. Corticosteroids, previously implicated as a 'trigger' for rheumatoid vasculitis, still forms the mainstay. D-Penicillamine, plasma exchange and a variety of cytotoxics all have roles. Cyclophosphamide is often used successfully to treat other forms of necrotising vasculitis such as polyarteritis, and on its own has been of value in rheumatoid disease. The immunosuppressive and clinical response may however take at least 10 days. More recent studies would suggest that the rational approach to treatment would be immediate use of anti-inflammatory drugs (high dose oral prednisolone or pulsed methylprednisolone), starting cyclophosphamide at the same time. Our patient certainly benefitted from this approach with dramatic healing of her ulcers, and halting of the progression of her neuropathy.

Comment

Acute rheumatoid vasculitis is rare but treatable. Early and aggressive therapy is vital. The present recommended regime is to treat with 'pulse' cyclophosphamide (e.g. 500 mg i.v. repeated weekly or fortnightly) in addition to oral corticosteroids in high dose initially and gradually tapering. Plasma exchange does not appear to provide additional help in the acute stage in our experience.

References

1. Scott D G I and Bacon P A. Intravenous cyclophosphamide plus methylprednisolone in the treatment of systemic rheumatoid vasculitis. *Am. J. Med.* 1984: **76**, 377–384
2. Winkelstein A, Starz T W and Agarawal A. Efficacy of combined therapy with plasmapheresis and immunosuppressants in rheumatoid vasculitis. *J. Rheumatol.* 1981: **11**, 162–166
3. Scott D G I, Bacon P A, Bothamley J E *et al.* Plasma exchange in rheumatoid vasculitis. *J. Rheumatol.* 1981: **8**, 433–439
4. Lakhanpal S, Conn D L and Lie J T. Clinical and prognostic significance of vasculitis as early manifestation of connective tissue disease syndromes. *Ann. Intern. Med.* 1984: **101**, 743–748

3.2 RHEUMATOID ARTHRITIS AND ANKLE SWELLING

History

Miss D.C. developed rheumatoid arthritis at the age of 29 and had to give up her job as a circus trapeze artist. Over the next 20 years her disease progressed with extensive joint destruction despite treatment with both penicillamine and gold, and by the time she was 40 years old she had been started on prednisolone. Over the next 5 years, the dose was reduced. She had a number of orthopaedic operations, including bilateral knee replacements, a right total hip replacement and bilateral excision of the metatarsal heads; but in general it was thought that her articular disease had burnt out.

At 48 she developed leg ulcers and noted that she was continually thirsty with stickiness of her eyes in the morning. Over that year her ankles began to swell and her GP noted the development of hepatomegaly. She began to lose weight and for the first time in the course of her disease developed rheumatoid nodules and a widespread purpuric vasculitic rash. She was cushingoid and had a rapid but small volume pulse with a blood pressure of 80/70 mmHg and 15 mm paradox. The JVP was elevated with prominent 'v' waves and the apex beat was impalpable with soft heart sounds on auscultation.

There was pitting oedema, but no evidence of active synovitis. Relevant investigations are listed:

Hb	10.4 g/L. normochromic normocytic
WC	normal
Platelets	normal
ESR	82 mm/h
ANA	positive (1:640)
Latex test	positive 1:320
Cryoglobulins	positive
Immune complexes	positive

X-ray showed widespread erosive joint disease, a pleural effusion and normal cardiac silhouette.

Progress and management

Despite the normal cardiac silhouette on chest X-ray, a diagnosis of constrictive pericarditis was pursued, and the presence of a large pericardial collection with poor ventricular function was confirmed by echocardiography. This, with her cutaneous vasculitis, suggested active rheumatoid disease and her prednisolone was increased to 20 mg daily and azathioprine introduced. This, along with percutaneous aspiration of 500 ml of fluid from the pericardial sac, failed to alter the physical signs. A pericardectomy was performed and a grossly thickened pericardium (5 mm thick) partially removed. She made a good recovery with return of her JVP and BP to normal and resolution of her ankle oedema. Her vasculitis responded well to the azathioprine and prednisolone.

Points for discussion

This woman illustrates that inactive joints do not necessarily reflect inactive rheumatoid disease. One year before her referral to hospital, her disease had changed its pattern, becoming systemic or 'malignant' with high titres of circulating immune complexes and cryoglobulinaemia, an important diagnostic pointer.

Pericarditis may not uncommonly complicate rheumatoid arthritis but often remains asymptomatic. Constrictive pericarditis is usually not associated with an effusion, although, as in this patient, fluid may be found. This complication may respond to medical treatment, but more often than not pericardectomy is required, and this should be done earlier rather than later.

Comment

For the practicing rheumatologist, two physical signs provide clinical lessons – one subtle and one obvious – chronic ankle oedema in an RA patient has a number of causes. So many of us have missed one possible diagnosis – chronic constrictive pericarditis.

She had developed a widespread purpuric vasculitic rash. Had this rash been confined to the lower limbs, its appearance, in a patient with rheumatoid arthritis complicated by a sicca syndrome, as occurred in our lady might suggest 'purpura hyperglobulinaemia', or the purpura might have been associated with the presence of cryoglobulinaemia, both conditions often complicating sicca syndrome, usually of the primary variety. On the other hand, widespread purpura in patients with rheumatoid disease can mean a 'change of gear' of rheumatoid disease which is generally accompanied by a more active immunological profile with positive C1q binding, high titres of rheumatoid factor and positive ANA.

References

1. Weismann M and Zvaifler N. Cryoglobulinaemia in rheumatoid arthritis. Significance in serum of patients with rheumatoid vasculitis. *Clin. Invest.* 1975: **56**, 725 – 739
2. Liss J P and Bachmann W T. Rheumatoid constrictive pericarditis treated by pericardectomy. *Arthritis Rheum.* 1970: **13**, 869 – 876
3. Thould A K. Constrictive pericarditis in rheumatoid arthritis. *Ann. Rheum. Dis.* 1986: **45**, 89 – 94

3.3   RHEUMATOID ARTHRITIS AND SHORTNESS OF BREATH

History

This 74-year-old man was diagnosed as having seropositive RA eighteen months previously. The polyarthritis, which came on acutely over a few days, affected his shoulders initially but then spread to involve other joints to a lesser degree. After an ineffective period on NSAIDs he was given a total of 450 mg of i.m. gold.

For two weeks prior to his hospital admission, he had complained of a productive cough (including several haemoptyses), accompanied by dyspnoea. The RA had worsened gradually at the same time.

Examination	Dyspnoeic at rest
	No clubbing, nodules, vasculitis, lymphadenopathy or splenomegaly
	Normotensive (120/70)
	Late inspiratory and expiratory crackles bilaterally
	Swelling of MCP joints, both hands
	Stiffness of shoulders and wrists

Investigations

Hb	10 g/L
WC	normal. No eosinophilia
Platelets	normal
ANA	positive (1:40)
RA latex test	positive (1:640)
Mantoux	negative
Schirmer's test	negative
Chest X-ray	Diffuse confluent alveolar shadowing of mid and lower zones, both lung fields
V/Q scan	Ill-defined defects in mid and lower zones
	No mismatch present
X-rays	Severe erosive polyarthropathy
Pulmonary function	Restrictive defect
	Impaired gas transfer
	Hypoxaemia

Lung biopsy	Severe fibrosing alveolitis
	Superimposed infection (purulent
	bronchopneumonitis)

Progress and management

Night sweats developed, accompanied by fever, with increasing shortness of breath while on the ward. Coarse crepitations extended into both mid-zones although the cough was still only minimally productive of white frothy sputum. His respiratory rate increased to 48/min.

Blood gases showed increasing hypoxaemia and he was placed on a combination of Septrin and cephalosporin. A sudden rapid deterioration in his condition required admission to the Intensive Care Unit requiring assisted ventilation. He died suddenly in respiratory failure.

| **Post-mortem** | Thrombotic non-infective endocarditis |
| **findings** | Diffuse interstitial fibrosis and bronchopneumonia |

Points for discussion

This patient illustrates several typical manifestations of RA

- An acute onset of polyarthritis affecting mainly the shoulders in elderly patients (particularly males).

- The appearance of interstitial fibrosis in this patient initially provoked a discussion on whether this was an example of gold lung or part of the rheumatoid process. Interstitial lung disease occurs in approximately 20–40% of RA patients and may or may not cause overt clinical symptoms. In a percentage of patients, the condition may be relatively acute with mean survival of less than 5 years similar to cryptogenic fibrosing alveolitis. There is a poor response to corticosteroid therapy. Some patients have responded to methotrexate, cyclophosphamide and azathioprine. Respiratory failure, pulmonary hypertension and cor pulmonale develop late in the disease.

- Fibrosing alveolitis has also been registered after treatment with gold (dosage varying from 175 to 1210 mg). The onset is usually sudden and usually manifests 12 weeks after commencement of therapy.

- Distinguishing points may be blood eosinophilia or other manifestations of gold hypersensitivity, e.g.   dermatitis
  thrombocytopaenia
  proteinuria.

- In both conditions clubbing is rare. Most patients respond to administration of steroids and withdrawal of the drug.

- Our case also illustrates the increased susceptibility of patients with RA to infection even in the absence of Sjögren's syndrome. Sudden deterioration of pulmonary function may be on this basis.

Comment

This man had seropositive and ANA-positive RA. While lung fibrosis is an occasional feature in such patients, the acuteness and severity was marked. Gold salts have been implicated in some cases of pulmonary fibrosis but our case illustrates the difficulty in establishing a cause-and-effect link.

References

1. Payne C R. Pulmonary manifestations of rheumatoid arthritis. *Br. J. Hosp. Med.* 1984: 192–197
2. Shiel W C and Prete P E. Pleuropulmonary manifestations of Rheumatoid Arthritis. *Semin. Arthritis Rheum.* 1984: 13, 235–242
3. Scott D L, Bradby G V H, Aitman T J *et al.* Relationship of gold and penicillamine therapy to diffuse interstitial lung disease. *Ann. Rheum. Dis.* 1981: 40, 136–141
4. Winterbauer R H, Wilske K R and Wheelis R F. Diffuse pulmonary injury associated with gold treatment. *N. Engl. J. Med.* 1976: 294, 919–921
5. Levinson M L, Lynch J P and Bower J S. Reversal of progressive, life-threatening gold hypersensitivity pneumonitis by corticosteroids. *Am. J. Med.* 1981: 71, 906–912

3.4 PULMONARY INVOLVEMENT: A RARE CAUSE

History

A 39-year-old woman with a twelve-year history of rheumatoid arthritis presented with exertional dyspnoea. The arthritis, which was severely deforming, had previously been treated with NSAIDs, antimalarials and intermittent courses of oral prednisolone. She had only recently developed Raynaud's phenomenon. She was a non-smoker and had never taken oestrogen-containing contraceptives.

On examination her arthritis was classical although there were no rheumatoid nodules. She was cyanosed, with an elevated JVP and marked pitting oedema of the ankles. There was a left parasternal heave, and a palpable P2 which was loud on auscultation with a pulmonary systolic murmur. There was no clinical evidence of pulmonary fibrosis.

Investigations

Hb	18.6 g/dl
PCV	56%
RA latex test:	positive (1:256)
ANA	negative
ENAs	negative

An ECG showed right axis deviation, and the CXR large proximal pulmonary arteries. A pulmonary angiogram was normal and the findings at right heart catheterization are shown in Table 3.4. Lung function tests were within normal limits.

Progress and management

The clinical diagnosis of pulmonary hypertension was confirmed by the invasive cardiac investigations described. The severe right heart failure initially responded to diuretics and she was anticoagulated to prevent pulmonary thrombotic episodes. Nifedipine did not produce any significant effect and she died 9 months later in severe right heart failure.

Table 3.4 Results of right heart catheterization

Pressures (mmHg)	Patient	NR (upper limit)
RA mean	14	5
RV	83/20	30/5
PA mean	49	20
PC	10	13
SA mean	91	100
Cardiac index	$1.3 \, \text{L min}^{-1} \text{m}^{-2}$	$2.5 - 3.5 \, \text{L min}^{-1} \text{m}^{-2}$

RA = Right atrium PA = Pulmonary artery RV = Right ventricle
PCW = Pulmonary capillary wedge SA = Systemic arterial pressure

Points for discussion

In this patient, pulmonary hypertension developed late in the course of her disease and in the absence of any definable parenchymal disease of the lungs. Other types of lung disease in patients with rheumatoid arthritis are:

1. Pleuritis (with or without effusions)
2. Pulmonary nodules
3. Pulmonary fibrosis
4. Pulmonary arteritis
5. Recurrent infections (especially associated with Sjögren's)
6. Pneumothorax (due to subpleural nodule rupture)

The development of pulmonary hypertension in rheumatoid arthritis is unusual and the condition is more typically seen in other connective tissue diseases, particularly systemic sclerosis, systemic lupus erythematosus or mixed connective tissue disease (MCTD). The paucity of reported cases reflects the rarity of this complication and where histology has been available, pulmonary arteritis is not infrequently seen. Often, however, the condition resembles the pulmonary hypertension seen in the primary 'idiopathic' variety with clear lung fields and no evidence of parenchymal lung disease or overt thromboembolism. The cause is unclear but it may result from prolonged arterial vasoconstriction in patients with hypereactive pulmonary vessels, and indeed a generalized vasospastic tendency may exist reflected by Raynaud's phenomenon, as in this patient. The eventual fatal outcome indicates inadequacies of available treatment.

Comment

Attempts are usually made to treat the two major mechanisms thought to be responsible for the development of pulmonary hypertension, i.e. vascular spasm, where drugs such as nifedipine may have a role (there may be a common underlying mechanism in patients with severe Raynaud's) and endarterial thrombosis, where anticoagulation might be a more logical treatment. Although primary thromboembolism or thrombosis *in situ* may be operating in a minority of patients, secondary thromboses occurring in vasoconstricted narrowed vessels have been shown to occur in patients with primary 'idiopathic' pulmonary hypertension.

References

1. Shiel W C and Prete P E. Pleuropulmonary manifestations of rheumatoid arthritis. *Semin. Arthritis Rheum.* 1984: **13**, 235 – 242
2. Asherson R A, Morgan S H, Hackett D *et al.* Rheumatoid arthritis and pulmonary hypertension. *J. Rheumatol.* 1985: **12**, 154 – 159
3. Hatano S and Strasser T (eds.) *Primary Pulmonary Hypertension.* Report of a WHO meeting 1975

3.5   DIARRHOEA AND WEIGHT LOSS

History

At the age of 14 years, Susan developed a juvenile chronic polyarthritis of the 'rheumatoid' type, with fever and profound anaemia. This remained active for years, despite treatment with prednisolone and attempts to control it with gold, D-penicillamine and cyclophosphamide – all withdrawn because of side effects. The arthritis left her with severe joint deformity although corrective orthopaedic surgery had been beneficial.

Fifteen years later, she was referred to hospital. Although still on low-dose prednisolone her arthritis had 'burnt' itself out. Her main complaint was of diarrhoea (4–9 times/day) and she had also started to lose weight. Two years before referral she had been treated for a bleeding duodenal ulcer which had been oversown, along with a vagotomy and pyloroplasty. On examination, she was pale and had marked thinning alopecia. The liver was just palpable but there was no splenomegaly. Neurological examination was normal. The results of a number of investigations are shown below.

Investigations

Hb	8.7 g/dl. hypochromic microcytic
WC	9.6×10^9/L. normal differential count
ESR	120 mm/h
Liver function	normal
Urea	16 mmol/L
Creatine	200 mcmol/L
Creatine clearance	35 ml/min
Proteinuria	2.3 g/24 h
Urinary sediment	normal
RA latex test	negative
ANA	negative

Progress and management

In view of the proteinuria and impaired renal function, a clinical diagnosis of systemic amyloidosis was made. A rectal biopsy was positive for amyloid staining, and a renal biopsy confirmed this as the cause of her renal disease. Since her rheumatoid disease was quiescent, further immunosuppressive therapy was not warranted. A ^{14}C breath test suggested bacterial overgrowth and this was confirmed by jejunal aspiration. Her diarrhoea came under control on tetracycline and antidiarrhoeal drugs, but her renal function continues to deteriorate.

Points for discussion

Although in this case the chronic diarrhoea may have been a complication of vagotomy and pyloroplasty, amyloidosis was the most likely diagnosis, with infiltration of the gut mucosa and secondary bacterial overgrowth, as was implied by the investigations. Amyloid neuropathy, although unusual in reactive amyloidosis, may be associated with autonomic dysfunction – another possible cause of diarrhoea.

Renal disease in amyloidosis occurs in 70–90% of patients and may be accompanied by an overt nephrotic syndrome, either as a direct result of glomerular deposition or from secondary renal vein thrombosis, especially if there are episodes of dehydration – the patient's diarrhoea being of particular relevance in this respect.

In patients with rheumatoid disease of more than 10 years duration, the diagnosis should be suspected if insidious proteinuria develops, if there is otherwise unexplained hepatosplenomegaly, or a rising ESR in the absence of active disease.

The diagnosis can only be positively confirmed by biopsy. A negative rectal biopsy does not exclude the diagnosis.

The prognosis is poor, though very variable.

Comment

Amyloid still haunts the patient with JCA. The advent of sensitive measurements of serum amyloid A (SAA) protein may, in time, predict an 'at risk' group of patients with persistently high SAA levels. Such patients might, for example, be considered for prophylactic colchicine treatment.

In the adult RA patient, there is a strong impression that amyloid is becoming a less frequent complication – indeed the majority of cases we have encountered during the past decade have been in patients with sero-negative arthritis and spondylitis, including adult Still's disease and long-standing psoriatic arthritis.

References

1. Hind R K, Baltz M and Pepys M B. Amyloidosis. *Med. Int.* 1984: **10**, 409–416
2. Glenner G G, Pinho E, Costa P and De Freitas F (eds.) *Amyloid and Amyloidosis.* 1980 (Amsterdam: Excerpta Medica)
3. Pasternack A, Ahonen J and Kuhlbck B. Renal transplantation in 45 patients with amyloidosis. *Transplantation*, 1986: **42**, 598–601

3.6   METHOTREXATE IN JOINT DISEASE

History

A 31-year-old housewife had been followed in the rheumatology clinic for ten years. Her symmetrical erosive polyarthritis had been particularly aggressive. She had been persistently seronegative for IgM rheumatoid factor, but in all other respects her disease was typical of rheumatoid arthritis.

Initially she had had a good response to sodium aurothiomalate (Myocrisin) but this had to be withdrawn because of severe oral ulcers. Subsequent courses of D-penicillamine and hydroxychloroquine had been ineffective. Prednisolone at a dose of 10 mg daily provided only minimal symptomatic improvement, and the addition of azathioprine contributed little. She had early morning stiffness in excess of two hours. Radiologically, her disease was progressing and she became housebound, finding it difficult even to look after her young son who coincidentally had developed Still's disease.

A variety of investigations mirrored the clinical evidence of disease activity.

Investigations

Hb	11.5 g/dl. normochromic normocytic
WC	$13.8 \times 10^9/L$
ESR	67 mm/h
RA latex test	negative
ANA	positive (1:40)
Immune complexes	positive by C1q and monoclonal rheumatoid factor binding assay (RFBA)

Progress and management

A maintenance dose of prednisolone was continued and oral methotrexate introduced in a total weekly dose of 7.5 mg, divided into 3 over 36 hours. Two months later there had been a dramatic improvement. Her morning stiffness had disappeared. She was coping much better with daily tasks, and her ESR fell to 16 mm/h with a rise in Hb. The methotrexate was withdrawn when she missed a period and feared pregnancy. There was a severe relapse of her arthritis which was 'recaptured' on reintroduction of the drug.

Points for discussion

The effectiveness of low-dose methotrexate in the treatment of the arthritis of psoriasis was described in the 1950s. Most of the guidelines for therapy were formulated within dermatology clinics and a once weekly pulsed regime was adapted to minimize toxicity. In the low doses used (7.5–15.0 mg weekly), bone marrow suppression seldom occurs. Minor side effects such as post-dose nausea, aphthous ulceration, dyspepsia and diarrhoea may be encountered but usually respond to dosage reductions and are seldom rated as severe by patients. An acute hypersensitivity pneumonitis has been rarely reported and usually resolves on withdrawal of methotrexate.

The major concern has been hepatic toxicity. A mild elevation of hepatocellular enzymes is often seen early in treatment and unusually a hypersensitivity hepatitis may occur. In the original psoriatic series, there was a 20% incidence of hepatic fibrosis on liver biopsy relative to cumulative dosage of 1 g or more. On this basis, a protocol of percutaneous liver biopsy pre-treatment and a 1.5 g cumulative dosage was recommended, particularly since abnormal blood LFTs correlate poorly with the incidence of fibrosis. However, with patient selection excluding those with a history of previous liver disease, obesity, diabetes mellitus and regular alcohol consumption, the incidence of hepatic fibrosis at follow-up biopsy was less than 10% at 2 years and limited to mild change only. Several centres have shown that it is rare for this fibrosis to progress to major cirrhosis despite continuing methotrexate therapy and no longer carry out liver biopsy.

Comment

There can be few more dramatic examples of an effective medication than the response to weekly methotrexate in many patients with aggressive synovitis. This drug is being increasingly accepted although the balance of therapeutic efficacy against long-term hazards is not yet known.

References

1. Gubner R, August S and Ginsburg V. Therapeutic suppression of tissue reactivity. II. Effect of aminopterin in rheumatoid arthritis and psoriasis. *Am. J. Med. Sci.* 1951: **221**, 176–182
2. Weinstein G C and Frost P. Methotrexate for psoriasis. A new therapeutic schedule. *Arch. Dermatol.* 1971: **103**, 33–38
3. Roenigk H H, Auenbach R, Maibach H I and Weinstein G D. Methotrexate guidelines revised. *J. Am. Acad. Dermatol.* 1982: **6**, 145–155
4. Kremer J M and Lee J K. Safety and efficacy of the use of methotrexate in longterm therapy for rheumatoid arthritis. *Arthritis Rheum.* 1986: **29**, 822–835
5. Wilkins R F, *et al.* Liver biopsies in patients on low dose pulse methotrexate for the treatment of rheumatoid arthritis. *Arthritis Rheum.* 1985: **28**, 577

3.7   AZATHIOPRINE IN RHEUMATOID ARTHRITIS

History

The patient, a 60-year-old causasian woman, first developed seropositive rheumatoid arthritis in 1967. A 3-year remission was obtained on sodium aurothiomalate (Myocrisin), but this was discontinued when an acute exfoliative dermatitis developed. A relapse soon occurred and D-penicill-amine was started, but this was stopped because of thrombocytopaenia (platelet count $< 100 \times 10^9$/L) which did not respond to dose reduction.

Progress and management

Prednisolone was introduced at a dose of 20 mg/day, and, although this controlled her symptoms well, she became cushingoid with recurrent 'flares' of arthritis if the dose was reduced below 10 mg/day. Azathioprine was introduced as a steroid-sparing agent at a dose of 150 mg/day (2.5 mg/kg) but stopped after 5 weeks because of nausea and vomiting. Her prednisolone was again increased because of a 'flare' and hydroxychloroquine added in an attempt to reduce steroid requirements. Again, a skin rash developed.

The patient developed severe oesophagitis with oesophageal ulceration at fibroscopy which healed on cimetidine. Her rheumatoid disease continued to progress and as a final attempt to reduce her steroid dependency, azathio-prine was reintroduced in a lower dose – 75 mg/day. After 2 – 3 months her disease had gone into remission and steroid therapy was successfully 'tailed off'.

Points for discussion

Patients with severe destructive rheumatoid arthritis commonly present a therapeutic problem. Steroids are often used in an attempt to minimize symptoms and keep the patient's day to day life tolerable. Often, such patients become steroid dependent and all attempts to introduce steroid-sparing agents fail.

We have often used azathioprine in this situation but its peak action is often only reached after 3 – 4 months. There may be haematological evidence of reduction in disease activity. Nausea and vomiting are frequent side effects but may be reduced by a temporary withdrawal of the drug and reintroduction at a lower dose, as in this patient. In fact, contrary to previous beliefs, some believe that azathioprine in low dosage (50–100 mg/day) is as effective as standard dose regimens, with fewer side effects, and should be considered for use in rheumatoid arthritis on a par with gold and penicillamine. Time will tell.

Comment

Azathioprine has come of age in RA, and most observers feel it has an important part to play in systemic or 'malignant' RA. Dyspepsia and abnormal liver function tests may be significant problems with the drug. Perhaps methotrexate has already overtaken it.

References

1. Urowitz M B, Hunter R, Bockman, A A H *et al.* Azathioprine in rheumatoid arthritis: a double blind study comparing full dose to half dose. *J. Rheumatol.* 1974: **1**, 274–281
2. Huskisson E C. Azathioprine. *Clin. Rheum. Dis.* 1984: **10**, 325–332

Section 4

THE VASCULITIDES

INTRODUCTION

'Vasculitis' is simply a descriptive term reflecting damage to blood vessel walls with inflammation and necrosis. This is seen in many of the connective tissue diseases, but is the the hallmark of a heterogeneous group of disorders, classified under the unifying diagnosis of 'systemic vasculitis' (Table 4.0).

Table 4.0 Classification of the vasculitides

Polyarteritis nodosa group [1]	–	Classical PAN
	–	Kawasaki's disease
	–	Hairy cell leukemia
Small vessel vasculitides [2]	**Granulomatous**	
	–	Wegener's granulomatosis
	–	Mid-line granulomatosis
	–	Churg – Strauss vasculitis
	Non – granulomatous	
	–	Hypersensitivity vasculitis
	–	Essential mixed cryoglobulinaemia
	–	Relapsing polychondritis
	–	Cogan's syndrome (vasculitis, nerve deafness and interstitial keratitis)
	–	Cutaneous vasculitis
	–	Behçet's disease
	–	Infective endocarditis
	–	Atrial myxoma
	–	Renal carcinoma
	–	Other connective tissue diseases
Giant cell arteritides [3]	–	Cranial arteritis
	–	Polymyalgia rheumatica
	–	Takayasu's disease
	–	Ankylosing spondylitis
	–	Reiter's disease

[1] Affect medium-sized arteries
[2] Affect arterioles and venules
[3] Affect large – medium arteries

90

Although the clinical spectrum is wide, they share two common features:

1. In most cases there are no specific serological tests, although in Wegener's granulomatosis and microscopic polyarteritis, the detection of antibodies against neutrophil cytoplasm looks encouraging.

2. The diagnosis, is therefore based on clinical findings, supported by tissue biopsy and arteriography. In many cases, the features may not be classical and diagnosis and treatment may therefore be unnecessarily delayed.

The lack of serological markers of disease activity may also make it difficult to decide when to discontinue treatment or reintroduce it in the face of a possible relapse.

In this section, we hope to illustrate just how heterogeneous a group these are, both in terms of clinical presentation and response to treatment.

Further reading

1. Fauci A J. Vasculitis. *J. Allergy Clin. Immunol.* 1983: 72, 211–233
2. Adu D, Howie A J, Scott D G I, Bacon P A, McGonigle R J S and Michael J. Polyarteritis and the kidney. *Q. J. Med.* 1987: **62**, 221–237
3. Savage C O J, Winearls C G, Evans D J, Rees A J and Lockwood C M. Microscopic polyarteritis: presentation pathology and prognosis. *Q. J. Med.* 1985: **56**, 467–483
4. Savage C O J, Winearls C G, Jones J, Marshall P D and Lockwood C M. Prospective study of radioimmunoassay for antibodies against neutrophil cytoplasm in diagnosis of systemic vasculitis. *Lancet* 1987: **1**, 1389–1393

4.1   STUFFY NOSE

History

At the age of 40, a military pilot developed mild asthma and irritating nasal congestion. He was referred for investigation by the ENT surgeons. Allergic rhinitis was diagnosed, and his symptoms were, to an extent, relieved by nasal polypectomy and sodium cromoglycate. Over the ensuing 5 years his asthma became more troublesome and he became generally unwell with malaise, weight loss, fever and migratory joint pains.

A year later he was admitted to hospital with bilateral nerve deafness, unilateral ptosis and a peripheral mononeuritis multiplex. On urinalysis he had both proteinuria and microscopic haematuria. Initial investigations are outlined below.

Investigations

Hb	15.8 g/dl
WC	14.9×10^9/L (30% eosinophilia)
ESR	18 mm/h
Creatinine clearance	60 ml/min
24 h urine protein	1.0 g

Liver function	
HBsAg	
ANA	
RA latex test	normal or negative
Immunoglobulins	
CXR	

Lung function tests	reversible bronchoconstriction

Progress and managment

A renal biopsy demonstrated a proliferative glomerulonephritis, with crescent formation in 4/20 glomeruli, and areas of fibrinoid necrosis. The systemic vasculitis was initially treated with high-dose prednisolone – 60 mg daily –

and cyclophosphamide. The fever resolved and no further neurological lesions developed. After a month the eosinophilia had disappeared. He remained on cyclophosphamide for a year. Attempts to withdraw the steroids were hampered by asthma. Although there had been no further neurological involvement, he was severely incapacitated by a right ulnar nerve palsy.

Points for discussion

In 1951 Churg and Strauss first documented a syndrome characterized by systemic vasculitis and hypereosinophilia in association with asthma and, more often than not, rhinitis. A strict histopathological diagnosis includes necrotizing vasculitis, extravascular granulomas and tissue infiltration with eosinophils, although the clinical pattern of the disease is usually sufficiently distinct to establish the diagnosis.

Hypertension is less frequently encountered than in PAN or Wegener's granulomatosis, but cardiac failure (eosinophilic cardiomyopathy) may complicate a proportion of cases. In common with the other vasculitides, immunological findings are usually unimpressive, although elevated IgE levels may be found in up to 50% patients.

As with PAN, there is an initial high morbidity stressing the need for early and aggressive treatment. As in this patient, asthma may be the only persisting, and often problematic, feature of the disease.

Comment

Why occasional patients with late-onset asthma and eosinophilia should suddenly 'change gear' and develop severe necrotizing vasculitis is a mystery. In a few anecdotal cases, the vasculitis is seemingly triggered by immunization or by desensitization 'shots'. Aggressive early treatment is mandatory. So far, follow-up of our cases reported some years ago has shown little tendency to recurrence.

References

1. Churg J and Strauss L. Allergic granulomatosis, allergic angiitis and polyarteritis nodosa. *Am. J. Pathol.* 1951: 27, 277–301
2. Lanham J, Elkon K, Pusey C and Hughes G R V. Systemic vasculitis with asthma and eosinophilia. A clinical approach to the Churg–Strauss syndrome. *Medicine (Baltimore)* 1984: 63, 65–81

4.2   HAEMOPTYSIS

History

In 1976, at the age of 26, a caucasian woman presented with superficial thrombophlebitis and erythema nodosum. During the following year she developed painful orogenital ulcers and was admitted to hospital with meningo-encephalitis and a focal retinal vasculitis. She complained of intermittent chest pain – pleuritic in character – and ventilation perfusion lung scans suggested pulmonary infarcts. She was anticoagulated and treated with a combination of prednisolone and cyclophosphamide.

Over the subsequent years, there were further severe disease flares. She became progressively short of breath on exertion and between 1981 and 1983 had several major haemoptyses.

Progress and management

A chest X-ray was performed, which revealed, not only a prominent pulmonary artery, but also a round opacity adjacent to the left hilum (Figure 4.2A). This had not been present on previous radiographs, and, in view of the prolonged treatment with immunosuppressive drugs, a malignant lesion was suspected.

Tomography (Figure 4.2B) was unhelpful. Ventilation/perfusion radio-nucleotide lung scans demonstrated multiple mismatched defects. Right heart catheterization confirmed pulmonary arterial hypertension (mean pressure 32 mmHg). Pulmonary angiography and CT scans of the thorax suggested that the perihilar mass was a sacculated and partially thrombosed aneurysm, arising at, or close to, the occluded origin of the apical branch of the left lower lobe artery. The haemoptyses continued, and bronchoscopy did not reveal an obvious source. A sudden massive haemoptysis followed resulting in death, and an aneurysm of the left lower lobe pulmonary artery was confirmed at post mortem, it having ruptured into its related bronchus.

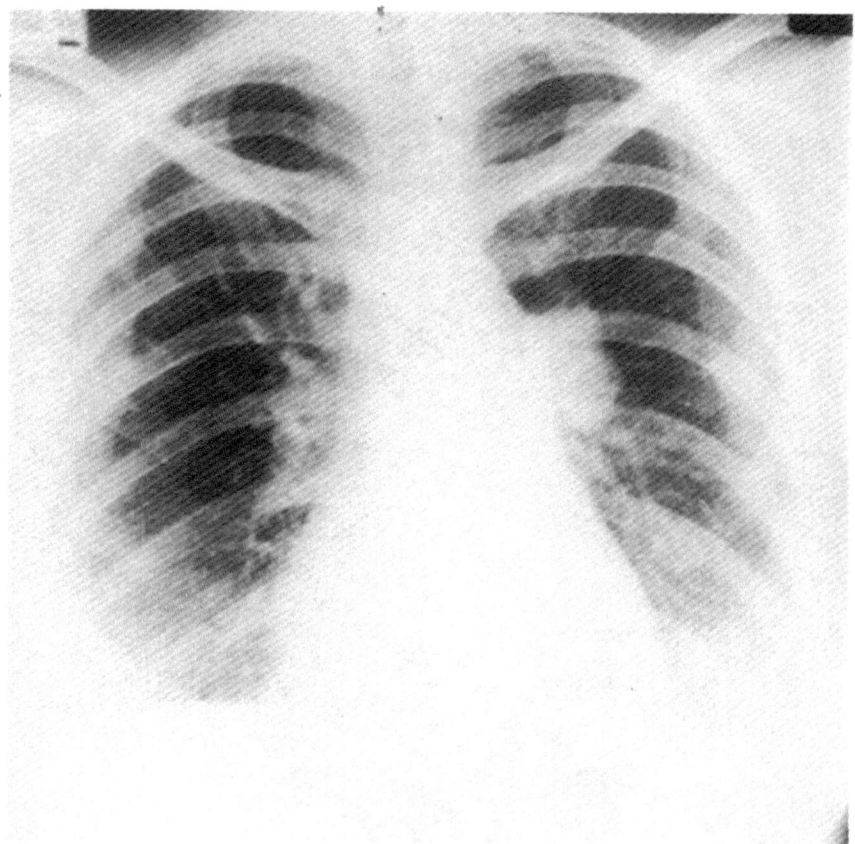

Figure 4.2A Plain chest radiograph showing rounded opacity adjacent to the left hilum (Reproduced from *Br. J. Radiol.* 1985: **58**, 79–80, by kind permission of the author and publishers)

Points for discussion

Pulmonary involvement is unusual in Behçet's, occurring in less than 5% of patients. Usually there is a diffuse non-specific vasculitis affecting arteries and veins of any calibre. The end result may be thrombosis, infarction, nodule formation, fibrosis, or cavitation, and consequently radiological changes may be extremely varied. Aneurysm formation is rare but does occur, so that investigations of radiographic pulmonary opacities in Behçet's should be as conservative as possible, and percutaneous biopsy considered with caution.

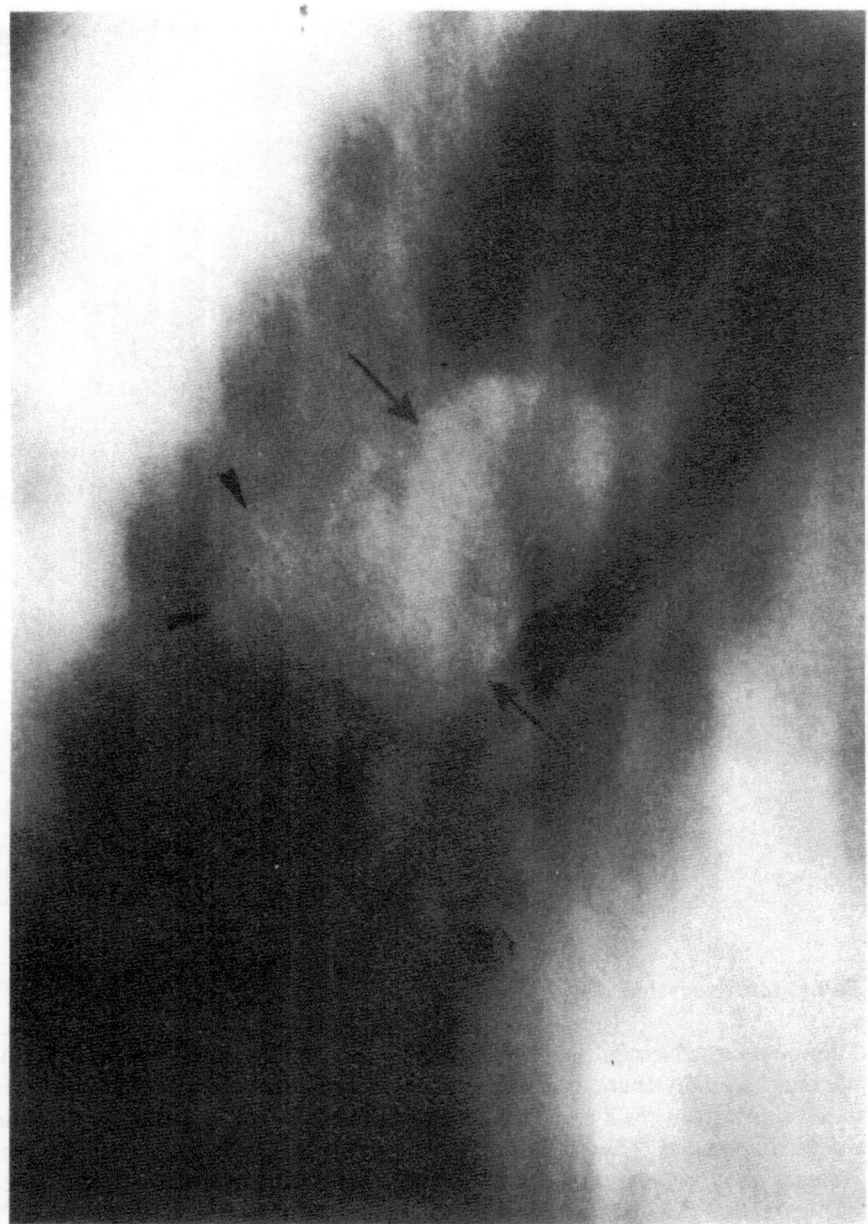

Figure 4.2B Lateral tomogram. A rounded opacity (arrowheads) lies immediately posterior to a prominent left pulmonary artery (arrows) (Reproduced from *Br. J. Radiol.* 1985: **58**, 79–80, by kind permission of the author and publishers)

Comment

The management of severe pulmonary vascular Behçet's is fraught with difficulty. New aneurysmal lesions often appear at the site of vascular surgical resection lines.

References

1. Shimizu T, Ehrlich G E, Inaba G and Hayashi K. Behçet's disease. *Semin. Arthritis Rheum.* 1979: **3**, 223-260
2. Cadman E C, Lundberg W B and Mitchell M S. Pulmonary manifestations of Behçet's syndrome. *Arch. Intern. Med.* 1976: **13**, 944-947
3. Gernier P, Bletry O, Cornud F, Goderu P and Nahum H. Pulmonary involvement in Behçet disease. *Am. J. Roentgenol.* 1981: **137**, 565-569
4. Efthimiou J, Johnston C, Spiro S G and Turner-Warwick M. Pulmonary disease in Behçet's syndrome. *Q. J. Med.* 1986: **58**, 259-280

4.3   DRUG-INDUCED DISEASE

History

Mr E S, a 70-year-old man, presented with a purpuric rash over both legs, becoming bullous at the ankles, with some ulceration. He had been unwell for two weeks with fever and an arthritis affecting his knees, ankles and elbows.

Ten years earlier he had had a myocardial infarct – cardiac failure had developed insidiously and had become increasingly resistant to conventional treatment. This had become so severe that a month prior to admission an angiotensin-converting enzyme (ACE) inhibitor had been started in addition to his long-term digoxin and diuretics.

Investigations

Hb	14.8 g/dl
WC	18.0×10^9/L neutrophilia
Platelets	normal
ESR	80 mm/h
Liver function	normal
Immunoglobulins	normal
ANA	
RA latex test	} negative
Cryoglobulins	

Progress and management

The arthritis settled with bed rest and a small dose of NSAIDs. The ACE inhibitor was withdrawn. The rash spread to involve the extensor aspects of both arms, and the lower limb ulcers extended (Figure 4.3). Biopsy of a fresh purpuric lesion revealed a leukocytoclastic vasculitis with IgA deposits on immunofluorescent staining.

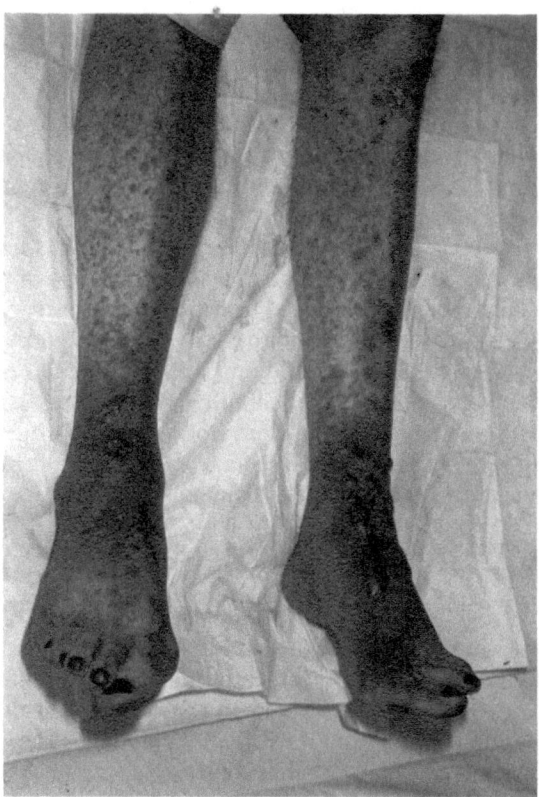

Figure 4.3 Cutaneous involvement in Schönlein – Henoch disease

He developed proteinuria, 2 g/24 h, with microscopic haematuria. Renal biopsy demonstrated a focal proliferative glomerulonephritis, again with IgA deposition. Despite normal renal function, prednisolone 40 mg daily was introduced. Two weeks after admission he had a melaena. He was transfused, but died three days later after a cardiac arrest.

Points for discussion

Schönlein – Henoch purpura is a vasculitic syndrome characterized by the involvement of skin, joints and gastrointestinal tract. Renal involvement is common. Bacterial infection, exposure to cold, insect stings, allergies, and a wide variety of drugs have all been incriminated. There is some evidence to support a role for IgA in pathogenesis, heavy deposits being found in the skin and in renal mesangium, and the renal histopathology is often indistinguishable from that seen in IgA neuropathy.

The disease is rare in adults, and the diagnosis should be regarded with suspicion until other causes of non-thrombocytopaenic purpura have been excluded – notably PAN, where immunofluorescent deposits are not usually seen in skin or renal biopsy specimens.

Although the data is sparse, the proportion of adults developing renal involvement is similar to that in childhood, with about 10% of patients having died from renal failure or needing renal transplant at 5 years.

Cutaneous reactions to ACE inhibitors are common, occurring in about 12% of patients. They are usually mild and self-limiting. To our knowledge, vasculitis has not been documented although 'lupus-like' syndromes have been described. Immunosuppression does not appear to affect the short- or long-term prognosis in Schönlein–Henoch syndrome – mortality being related to renal or gastro-intestinal involvement, as in this case.

Comment

Chronic leg ulcers and purpura in the middle-aged are often the presenting symptoms of a vasculitis. PAN, essential mixed cryoglobulinaemia and primary Sjögren's should be considered in the differential diagnosis in the absence of clear-cut rheumatoid arthritis. Schönlein–Henoch syndrome represents an unusual cause of this clinical picture.

References

1. Roth D A, Wilz D R and Theil G B. Schönlein–Henoch syndrome in adults. *Q. J. Med.* 1985: **55**, 145–152
2. Cameron J S. The nephritis of Schönlein–Henoch purpura. In *Current Problems in Progress in Glomerulonephritis* 1979: 283–309 (Wiley)
3. Goodfield M J and Millard L G. Severe cutaneous reaction to Captopril. *Br. Med. J. (Clin. Res.)* 1985: **290**, 111
4. Ace inhibitors: Enalapril and Captopril compared. *Drugs Ther. Bull.* 1985: **23**, 89–91

4.4   POST-PUERPERAL HEADACHE

History

A month after delivery of her first child, a 24-year-old woman developed frontal headaches, sore eyes and nasal stuffiness. She felt unwell and consulted her GP who prescribed a course of antibiotics.

Her condition deteriorated and she complained of nocturia and ankle swelling. She was admitted to her local hospital with fever and splinter haemorrhages in the nail beds. There was a persistent tachycardia and diastolic hypertension.

Investigations

Hb	8.4 g/dl. normochromic normocytic
WC	13.4 x 10^9/L neutrophilia
ESR	142 mm/h
Renal function	normal
Alkaline phosphatase	805 IU/L
Other liver function tests	normal
ANA	
RA latex test	
Immunoglobulins	all normal or negative
Complement studies	
Cryoglobulins	

Progress and management

A CXR showed a rounded opacity in the right lower lobe. Blood cultures were persistently sterile and an echocardiogram was normal. Nonetheless, she was treated with intravenous antibiotics but failed to improve. A systemic vasculitis was suspected and high-dose steroids introduced. Although the fever and tachycardia resolved, she developed collapse of the bridge of her nose (Figure 4.4) and a peripheral neuropathy. She was transferred to our unit for advice and further management. A renal biopsy, performed because of persisting haematuria and proteinuria, and deteriorating renal function,

101

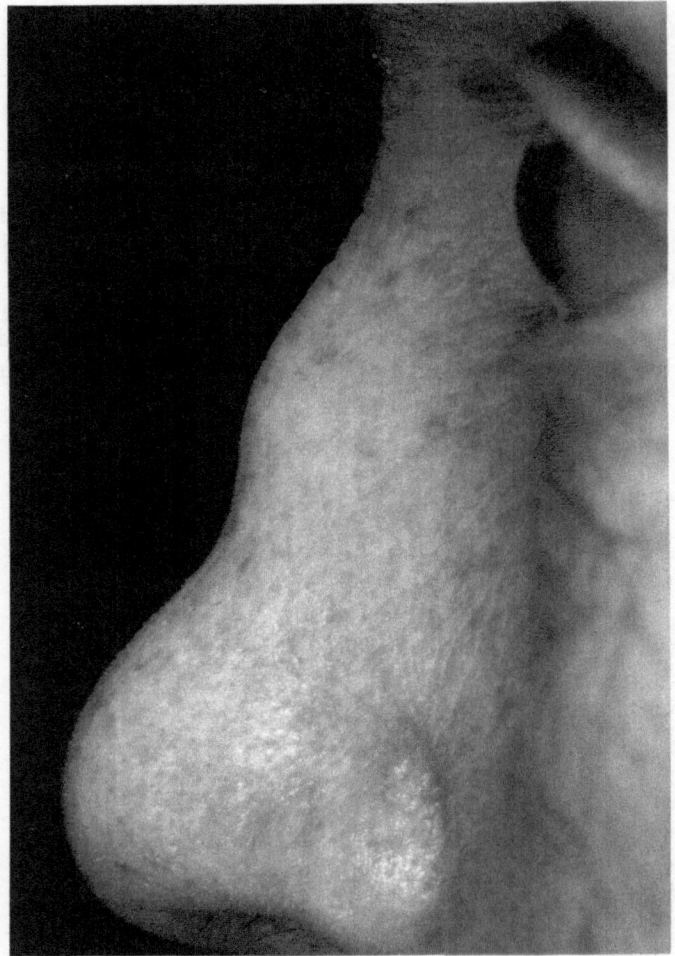

Figure 4.4 Collapse of nasal cartilage

demonstrated a focal proliferative glomerulonephritis with widespread crescent formation and necrosis, typical of Wegener's granulomatosis. The prednisolone was continued and intravenous cyclophosphamide introduced. She was discharged on a combination of prednisolone and oral cyclophosphamide with slow improvement although her renal function remained impaired.

Points for discussion

Although granulomata were never demonstrated, we believe this patient represents a clear case of Wegener's granulomatosis with mid-line nasal necrosis and collapse, lung infiltrates, nephritis, neuritis and a neutrophilia, with evidence of necrosis on renal biopsy.

Onset, or exacerbation of disease in pregnancy or the puerperium, is well recognized in SLE, but is not regarded as a feature of other vasculitic illnesses, although this case and others would suggest that the hormonal and immunological changes associated with pregnancy may precipitate such an onset in susceptible individuals.

Wegener's granulomatosis was considered a rapidly fatal disease, although the prognosis has been considerably improved since the introduction of cyclophosphamide. The outlook, however, must still be guarded, as indicated by a recent study from this hospital where the three-year survival was only 45%.

Comment

Experience with Wegener's granulomatosis has taught us a number of lessons.

1. The disease often progresses dramatically if the diagnosis is strongly suspected. Do not necessarily wait for histology.
2. Steroids alone are inadequate. Cyclophosphamide (preferably i.v.) is mandatory.
3. The histology often shows only necrosis and no granulomata.

References

1. Talbot S F, Man D M and Levinton A J. Wegener's granulomatosis: first report of a case with onset during pregnancy. *Arthritis Rheum.* 1984: 27, 109 – 112
2. Pinching A J, Lockwood C M, Pussell B A, Rees A J, Sweeney P, Evans D J, Bowley N and Peters D K. Wegener's Granulomatosis, observations on eighteen patients with severe renal disease. *Q. J. Med.* 1983: 52, 435 – 460
3. Fauci A S, Hanes B F, Katz P, Wolff S M. Wegener's granulomatosis. Prospective clinical and therapeutic experience with 85 patients for 21 years. *Ann. Intern. Med.* 1983: 98, 76 – 85

4.5   ESSENTIALLY MAD

History

J.E., a 56-year-old Polish refugee, was referred to the rheumatology unit when he developed a purpuric rash over both lower limbs (Figure 4.5). He had consulted his general practitioner over the past year complaining of aching in both joints and muscles. His wife claimed that there had been some episodes when he had become confused and aggressive at home, and that there had been a marked deterioration in his memory and ability to concentrate. Additional findings on examination included hepatosplenomegaly and some periungual infarcts. There were no focal neurological signs, but both short- and long-term memory were impaired and he was clearly disorientated in time and place.

Progress and management

Investigations revealed impaired renal function with a creatinine clearance of 25 ml/min and evidence of active nephritis on examination of the urinary sediment. The full blood count and clotting studies were normal. He had hypergammaglobulinaemia and a heavy cryoprecipitate (5 g/dl). This contained polyclonal IgG and monoclonal IgM with rheumatoid factor activity. A diagnosis of essential mixed cryoglobulinaemia was made. Initial treatment with plasma exchange was followed by high-dose prednisolone and intravenous cyclophosphamide. His general condition did not improve and he died following a massive haematemesis.

Points for discussion

The purpura – myalgia – cryoglobulinaemia syndrome was first described by Meltzer and colleagues in 1966, the cryoprecipitates containing 19S and 7S proteins. The cryoglobulinaemia is of a mixed type in that it usually contains immunoglobulins of at least two classes. More often than not, one of the immunoglobulins is IgM with rheumatoid factor (anti-IgG) activity.

Subsequent studies in this group of patients showed that almost three quarters of the cases had HBsAg antibody activity, and it suggested that the syndrome may reflect persisting hepatitis infection.

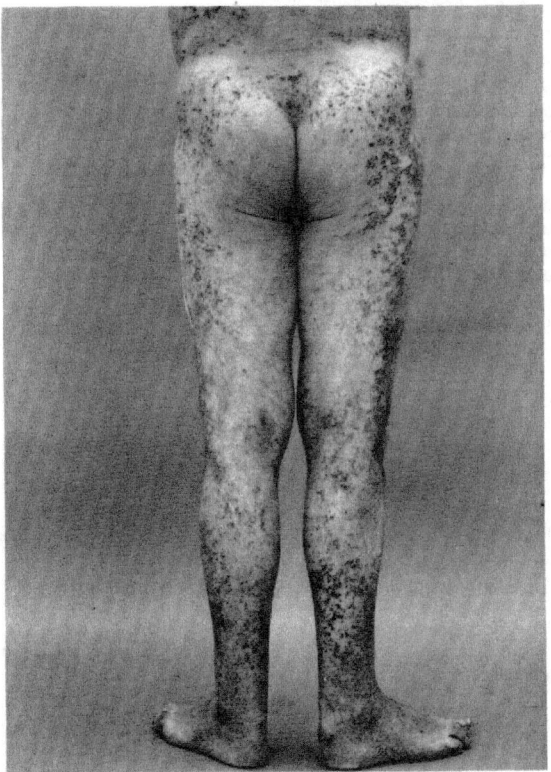

Figure 4.5 Gravitational purpura in mixed essential cryoglobulinaemia

Secondary mixed cryoglobulinaemia may complicate a variety of conditions, including most of the connective tissue diseases, most serious infections, in particular endocarditis, and chronic liver and bowel diseases. A classification of cryoglobulinaemia is suggested in Table 4.5.

Comment

Mixed cryoglobulinaemia is an important diagnosis to make – it is very treatable, yet potentially fatal, as shown in this case. The careful taking of blood at 37°C, allowing it to clot and leaving the serum at 4°C for 2 days is one of the simplest and cheapest tests in medicine.

105

Table 4.5 A classification of cryoglobulinaemias

Unmixed (monoclonal)
        Associated with myeloma
        Associated with lymphoma
        Associated with Waldenström's macroglobulinaemia
        Essential

Mixed (rheumatoid factor – IgG complexes)
(a) **With polyclonal rheumatoid factors**
        Associated with chronic inflammatory/infectious disease
        Associated with autoimmune disease (especially Sjögren's)
        Essential
(b) **With monoclonal rheumatoid factors**
        Associated with lympho – myeloproliferative disease
        Essential

References

1. Meltzer M, Franklin E C, Elias K, McCluskey R T and Cooper N. Cryoglobulinaemia – a clinical and laboratory study. *Am. J. Med.* 1966: 40, 837–856
2. Brouet J C, Clauvel J P, Danon F, Klein M and Seligmann M. Biological and clinical significance of cryoglobulins, a report of 86 cases. *Am. J. Med.* 1974: 57, 775–788
3. Gharavi A E, Campion C T and Hughes G R V. Use of anti-idiotypic antibodies to demonstrate rheumatoid factor producing bone marrow cells in essential mixed cryoglobulinaemia. *Ann. Rheum. Dis.* 1984: 43, 651–652

4.6   IN SEARCH OF A DIAGNOSIS

History

A 33-year-old teacher first developed severe non-migrainous headaches in 1983. These started shortly after a six-week episode of bloody diarrhoea associated with weight loss.

Three months later she was admitted under our care with fever, bilateral scleritis and bilateral nerve deafness. There were a few small mouth ulcers. There was some fine nystagmus on lateral gaze, and mild gait ataxia. Clinical examination was otherwise normal. Urinalysis was also normal.

Investigations

Hb	13.5 g/dl
WC	34.0×10^9/L
Platelets	800×10^9/L
ESR	79 mm/h
CRP	95 mcg/ml
Renal function	normal
Liver function	normal
ANA	negative
RA latex test	negative
Immune complexes	negative
Cryoglobulins	negative

Progress and management

A clinical diagnosis of systemic vasculitis was made and high-dose steroids started. Surprisingly, a 6 g IgA paraprotein was detected with trace Bence Jones proteinuria. Examination of the marrow was, however, normal, as was a skeletal survey. Visceral angiography did not demonstrate any features of PAN. The nodular scleritis resolved and there was some improvement in her deafness and balance.

The steroid dose was gradually reduced, and she was readmitted six months later with deafness and vertigo. She had bilateral ocular pain and large central scotomata with evidence of severe papillitis. Within a few hours, vision in the left eye was lost. Protein electrophoresis confirmed persistence of the paraprotein and she was treated with plasma exchange, pulsed methylprednisolone and cyclophosphamide. There was dramatic improvement although she remains blind in the left eye.

In view of diarrhoea as the presenting symptom, investigations to exclude inflammatory bowel disease were performed. These were all normal, except for a small bowel enema which showed some ileal nodularity. A CT scan suggested some enlarged para-aortic abdominal nodes. These were biopsied at laparotomy. There was no evidence of lymphoma.

Points for discussion

This patient is a perfect illustration of how difficult things can be when the presenting features and investigations do not fall into a succinct diagnostic category. The illness was obviously vasculitis – largely confined to the cranial nerves. There was no renal involvement and no evidence of PAN angiographically. Cogan's syndrome, a variant of PAN, may present with ataxia and nerve deafness, but is usually associated with interstitial keratitis.

Benign paraproteins have been described in association with connective tissue diseases, particularly RA and SLE, but only rarely. Paraproteinaemia and cryoglobulinaemia are well documented in association with malignancies, particularly lymphoma.

Overall, in vasculitis, neurological involvement is frequent, occurring in 40% of patients. Prompt introduction of cyclophosphamide is recommended and may prevent long-term sequelae in such patients.

Comment

This patient – 3 years on – is doing well on low dosage prednisolone alone. As the diagnosis is imperfect, the outlook must be equally uncertain.

References

1. Cogan D G. Syndrome of non-syphilitic interstitial keratitis and vestibuloauditory symptoms. *Arch. Ophthalmol.* 1945: 33, 144
2. Rubin L, Urowitz M and Prunzanski W. Systemic lupus erythematosus with paraproteinaemia. *Arthritis Rheum.* 1984: 27, 638–644
3. Moore P M and Cupps T R. Neurological complications of vasculitis. *Ann. Neurol.* 1983: 14, 155–167
4. Moore P M and Fauci A S. Neurological manifestations of systemic vasculitis. A retrospective and prospective study of the clinico-pathologic features and response to therapy. *Am. J. Med.* 1981: 71, 517–524

4.7   SPOTS BEFORE THE EYES

History

In 1978 a 36-year-old woman presented to her local hospital with crops of pink papules with an atrophic white centre over the trunk and extremities. Initially these caused some diagnostic confusion, but subsequently a diagnosis of Degos' disease was made.

In 1980 she developed an ischaemic myelopathy and in 1982 had a central retinal artery occlusion and bilateral choroidal infarcts. Over the next year she had multiple further neurological episodes, including ataxia, dysphasia and bladder incontinence.

Investigations

Hb	normal
WC	normal
Platelets	normal
ESR	40 mm/h
RA latex test	negative
VDRL	positive (TPHA negative)
Prothrombin time	prolonged
ANA	negative
ENAs	negative
Lupus anticoagulant	present
Antibodies to cardiolipin	medium positive (IgG)

Progress and management

She was treated with prednisolone and azathioprine and given intermittent pulses of cyclophosphamide. The anticardiolipin antibody levels remained elevated. She developed a further spinal cord lesion at C8 which eventually led to her death.

Points for discussion

Kohlmeir and Degos described a condition known as malignant atrophic papulosis (Degos' disease) in the 1940s. It was usually fatal as a result of multiple bowel perforations or more unusual widespread CNS vascular lesions. Pathologically there is primarily involvement of the arteriolar intima with endothelial proliferation and occlusion.

The association between anticardiolipin antibodies, the lupus anticoagulant and a tendency to thrombosis is well known. Anticardiolipin antibodies were found in 13/15 patients with SLE and cerebral infarction – differing significantly from control groups. It is difficult to ignore the possible aetiological implications of anticardiolipin antibodies in this patient and their potential use in directing and monitoring treatment of such a fatal disease.

Comment

The recent discovery that anticardiolipin antibodies are strongly associated with thrombosis has opened new perspectives in vascular diseases. The association appears to be particularly strong in non-inflammatory 'vasculopathies' and may provide useful information in such diverse conditions as multiple DVTs, recurrent strokes, early myocardial infarction and recurrent placental thrombosis with recurrent abortion. Measurement of anticardiolipin antibodies may provide guidance as to when anticoagulation can be stopped.

References

1. Degos R, Delort J and Tricot R. Dermatite papulosquameuse atrophiante. *Bull. Soc. Franc. Dermatol. Syph.* 1942: **49**, 148–150
2. Dastur D R, Singal B S and Shroff H J. CNS involvement in malignant atrophic papulosis, vasculopathy and coagulopathy. *J. Neurol. Neurosurg. Psychiatr.* 1981: **44**, 156–160
3. Boey M L, Colaco C B, Gharavi A E, *et al.* Thrombosis in SLE. A striking association with the presence of circulating lupus anticoagulant. *Br. Med. J.* 1983: **287**, 1021–1023
4. Hughes G R V. The anticardiolipin syndrome. *Clin. Exp. Rheumatol.* 1985: **3**, 285–286
5. Harris E N, Gharavi, A E, Asherson R A *et al.* Cerebral infarction in systemic lupus erythematosus – association with anticardiolipin antibodies. *Clin. Exp. Rheumatol.* 1984: **2**, 47–51

4.8   TB OR NOT TB

History

A 23-year-old Vietnamese girl was admitted to her local hospital with a short history of a non-productive cough and fever. A plain chest radiograph was normal, as was sputum examination for tubercule. A Mantoux test was strongly positive, and, because of a high index of suspicion, antituberculous chemotherapy was started.

Her fever and cough did not settle and she developed recurrent episodes of haemoptysis. At bronchoscopy, some granulomatous lesions were seen on both cords and there was evidence of diffuse mucosal inflammation. Aspirates and biopsies were taken.

Progress and management

During the night she developed stridor and became acutely dyspnoeic and required an emergency tracheostomy. A specimen of tracheal cartilage taken at the time subsequently showed histological evidence of polychondritis. High-dose prednisolone was started with resolution of her fever, although she remained breathless and subject to recurrent chest infections.

She produced some early photographs of herself (Figure 4.8). There had quite clearly been some nasal collapse, even though this must have been gradual and painless. She was also tender over her sternoclavicular cartilages. Lung function tests were markedly obstructive and pulmonary tomography showed extensive bronchial stenosis. Slit lamp examination of the eyes, echocardiography and urinalysis were all normal.

Apart from a mild anaemia, raised ESR and polyclonal hypergammaglobulinaemia, investigations were all normal. Specific assays for anticartilage antibodies were positive. The patient became a difficult management problem in that, although there was no evidence of further cartilaginous damage, she became steroid-dependent with diffuse joint pain and increased dyspnoea on steroid withdrawal. Azathioprine was added as a 'steroid-sparing' agent.

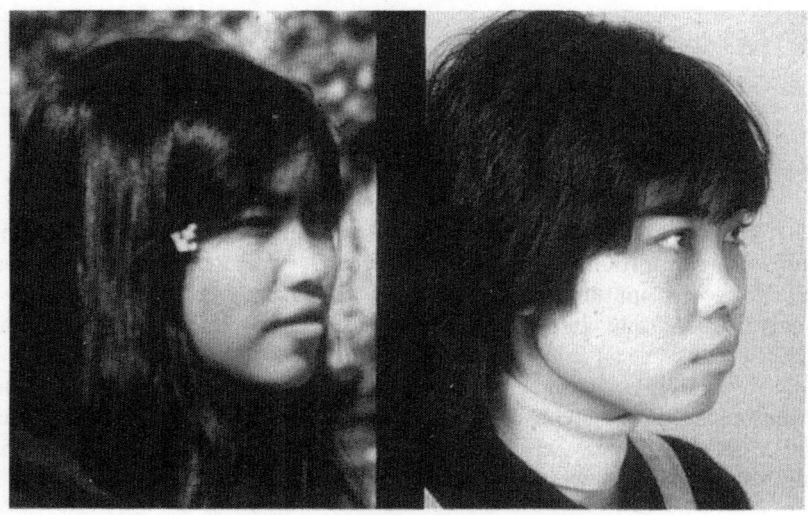

Figure 4.8 Change of nasal contour in patient

Points for discussion

Relapsing polychondritis is an unusual condition which primarily affects the mucopolysaccharide component of cartilage ground substance, resulting in inflammation and weakening of cartilage. Inflammation of the pinna, although classically described, occurs infrequently. Nasal collapse occurs more often, eventually in 75% of patients, and may not always be obvious, as in this case. The differential diagnosis is between Wegener's granulomatosis, syphilis, sarcoidosis and secondary collapse which occurs rarely in SLE and other connective tisssue diseases.

Involvement of the cartilage of the respiratory tract is serious and predisposes to infection, one of the commonest causes of death in this disease.

An arthritis, usually 'seronegative' in distribution, is often seen. Involvement of the aorta and aortic valves is unusual but has been reported.

Comment

Chondritis is a symptom complex found either in isolation (polychondritis) or during excerbations of certain diseases, particularly Wegener's granulomatosus and the connective tissue diseases.

Although some cases progress irrevocably to tracheal and bronchial collapse, in other cases the disease appears to be self limiting.

References

1. Michet C J, McKenna C H, Luthra H S and O'Fallow W M. Relapsing polychondritis. Survival and predictive role of early disease manifestations. *Ann. Intern. Med.* 1986: **104**, 74 – 78
2. O'Hanlan M, McAdam L P, Bluestone R and Pearson C M. The arthropathy of relapsing polychondritis. *Arthritis Rheum.* 1976: **19**, 191 – 194

4.9   A VISIT TO LOURDES

History

In 1965, this 29-year-old woman spent five months in hospital with an illness presenting with rash, fever, anaemia and a polyarthritis. A diagnosis of rheumatoid arthritis was made and she was treated with aspirin.

Five years later she represented with episodes comprising a transient maculopapular rash, intermittent high fever and a symmetrical polyarthritis principally affecting the wrists, knees and cervical spine. She was examined by Prof. Eric Bywaters and a diagnosis of 'adult' Still's disease was made.

Progress and management

Over the ensuing years, she was treated with a variety of therapeutic agents including:

Steroids in a variety of forms
NSAIDs
Azathioprine
Gold
D-Penicillamine
Sodium cromoglycate

These had little impact on the episodes of disease which continue to punctuate and incapacitate her life. During a recent and aggressive flare of disease, associated with weight loss and marked constitutional upset, non-allergic diets were tried – again with little impact. She made a pilgrimage to Lourdes.

Points for discussion

Patients with adult Still's disease often present a diagnostic dilemma. The condition is so named because of its resemblance to systemic-onset juvenile arthritis (JCA). The diagnosis is clinical and based on the following triad of features:

114

Rash   a salmon pink, evanescent maculopapular eruption, usually confined to the trunk and proximal limbs. It is non-pruritic, comes and goes with the fever, and is usually evident in the late afternoon, often associated with dermatographia.

Fever   typically high and spiking usually in the evening with brief duration.

Arthritis   usually affecting larger joints and, in particular, the wrists, where erosive disease usually results in carpal ankylosis. A particular feature is neck pain which may be myalgic in origin.

Histologically, the rash reflects a small-vessel vasculitis on which the disease is based. Lymphadenopathy and splenomegaly may occur, as may a serositis. Apart from normochromic normocytic anaemia and raised ESR, laboratory abnormalities are unusual. In common with other vasculitides, thrombocytosis and raised alkaline phosphatase are sometimes seen.

Long-term follow up of our original patients confirms the distinctive nature of the syndrome. Men are probably affected as often as women. Almost all patients had had a relapsing course lasting more than 20 years, and all had developed carpal ankylosis. The MCP joints were spared, but 50% had radiological evidence of DIP involvement. All patients had remained latex negative, and, even during relapses, immune complexes were never detected. Unusually, in comparison with JCA, only one patient had developed systemic amyloidosis. An aetiological basis for this unusual disease remains elusive.

Comment

Look at the wrists – in most patients referred, the investigation of prolonged high fever centres on the exclusion of lymphoma or very chronic infection. However, very few diseases other than adult Still's give a history of years of high fever with little to show other than stiffness of the wrists and neck.

Although the disease is not life-threatening, the treatment is often unsatisfactory.

References

1. Bywaters E G L. Still's disease in the adult. *Ann. Rheum. Dis.* 1971: **30**, 121–133
2. Elkon K B, Hughes G R V, Bywaters E G L *et al.* Adult onset Still's disease. Twenty year follow-up and further studies of patients with active disease. *Arthritis Rheum.* 1982: **25**, 647–654
3. Larson E B. Adult Still's disease. Evolution of a clinical syndrome and diagnosis, treatment and follow-up of 17 patients. *Medicine (Baltimore)* 1984: **63**, 82–91
4. Wouters J M G W and van de Putte L B A. Adult onset Still's; clinical and laboratory features, treatment and progress of 45 cases. *Q. J. Med.* 1986: **61**, 1055–1065
5. Cush J J, Medsger T A, Christy W C, Herbert D C and Cooperstein L A. Adult onset Still's disease: clinical course and outcome. *Arthritis Rheum.* 1987: **30**, 186–194

4.10   PSEUDO-SECONDARIES IN VASCULITIS

History

Mrs P. presented, aged 59, to her referring hospital with a two-month history of ill health beginning with bilateral otitis media and deafness resistant to several courses of antibiotics. Subsequently, she experienced intermittently red eyes and epistaxis. One month after the initial symptoms she developed a cough with haemoptysis accompanied by rapid weight loss of one stone in six weeks, intense malaise and recurrent fevers. There was no past history of ear or sinus infections.

Her chest X-ray showed right middle lobe consolidation and 'multiple opacities'. She was thought to have a secondary malignancy but extensive investigation proved normal. Attention was then re-focused on her head and neck symptoms and a nasal mucosal biopsy was performed which revealed necrotizing granuloma. By this time her renal function had deteriorated considerably, having been normal at presentation. A diagnosis of Wegener's granulomatosis was made and she was commenced on prednisolone 60 mg/day by mouth and referred for our opinion.

Examination revealed an ill woman who was febrile, anaemic and deaf with bilateral episcleritis and signs of right middle lobe consolidation. There were no clinical abnormalities detectable in the gastrointestinal or neurological systems.

Investigation

Hb	11.2 g/dl. normochromic normocytic
WC	15.6×10^9/L (neutrophil leukocytosis)
ESR	112 mm/h
Creatinine	317 mcg/L
Sputum culture	negative
Blood culture	negative
Chest X-ray	unchanged
Urinalysis	1–2 + proteinuria

Progress and management

In view of the marked deterioration in her renal function, it was decided to treat her with weekly pulses of intravenous cyclophosphamide (500 mg). Over the next three weeks her deafness improved. Her epistaxis and haemoptysis ceased and her malaise lessened. Changes in her chest X-ray lagged behind the clinical improvement, and indeed fluffy consolidation waxed and waned in the absence of any change in her physical signs over this period. Her treatment was changed to oral cyclophosphamide 100 mg/day and prednisolone was tapered off over the ensuing weeks.

Outpatient follow-up three months later showed a virtual clearing of her chest X-ray, white cell count fell to 6.7 x 10^9/L, and ESR dropped to 40 mm/h. She had some residual deafness and effort intolerance (in part due to steroid myopathy) but was otherwise well.

Comment

There are various subsets of inflammatory arteritis, including Wegener's, Churg–Strauss, vasculitis with otitis media, etc.

A clinical lesson which comes from experience of these cases is the importance of a history of ENT symptoms (deafness, sinusitis, etc.) in *any* or *all* of the variants.

References

1. Fauci A S, Haines B F, Katz P and Wolff S M. Wegener's granulomatosis: Prospective clinical and therapeutic experience with 85 patients for 21 years. *Ann. Intern. Med.* 1983: **98**, 76–85
2. Kovarsky J. Clinical pharmacology and toxicology of cyclophosphamide: Emphasis on use in rheumatic diseases. *Semin. Arthritis Rheum.* 1983: **12**, 359–372

Section 5

POLYMYOSITIS

INTRODUCTION

The incidence of myositis is reported as 0.5/100 000, women being affected more frequently than men (3:1). The clinical classification remains controversial, although that of Bohan and Peter remains the most acceptable (Table 5.0).

Myositis may complicate other connective tissue diseases, such as SLE, scleroderma and MCTD, but it is worth mentioning that patients with 'primary' PM/DM often have some 'overlap' features, the disease being preceded or complicated by a mild synovitis or tendinitis, as in patient 5.2. Raynaud's phenomenon can be marked and there may be subclinical or overt Sicca syndrome. Indeed, it is this particular group of patients that appear to be at risk of developing pulmonary fibrosis – accompanied by anti-Jo-1 antibody detectable in their serum as in case 5.2. A proportion of patients initially diagnosed as primary PM/DM may progress to true scleroderma.

The diagnosis of myositis is confirmed by:

Elevated serum muscle enzymes, usually AST, CPK, LHD or aldolase, although any one may be normal, even in acute disease;

Electromyography (EMG) with fibrillation, polyphasic action potentials and repetitive high-frequency discharges;

Muscle biopsy – although disease involvement is often patchy and negative biopsies can be obtained.

The large majority of patients are steroid responsive, the patients being seen in our unit usually representing treatment failures or the more unusual or complicated. Steroid-resistant disease has a high morbidity and mortality and aggressive or 'experimental' treatment in such patients, we feel is justified. The use of total body irradiation, antilymphocyte globulin and cyclosporin A has been explored. Muscle enzyme levels have, in the past, formed the cornerstone of monitoring response to treatment, but they may sometimes be misleading (patient 5.1), and, in conjunction with our physiotherapy department, we have found strain gauge myometry an indispensible tool in assessing response to treatment or deterioration.

Table 5.0 Clinical classification of myositis

GROUP 1	Primary idiopathic polymyositis
GROUP 2	Primary idiopathic dermatomyositis
GROUP 3	Malignancy-associated myositis
GROUP 4	Childhood dermatomyositis/polymyositis
GROUP 5	Dermatomyositis/polymyositis associated with other connective tissue diseases (e.g. MCTD, SLE)

References

1. Bohan A and Peter J B. Polymyositis and dermatomyositis. *N. Engl. J. Med.* 1975: 292, 344–347
2. Edwards R H T, Isenberg D A, Wiles C M *et al.* The investigation of inflammatory myopathy. *J. R. Coll. Phys.* 1981: 15, 19–24
3. Edwards R H T and McConnel M. Hand held dynamometer for evaluation of voluntary muscle functions. *Lancet* 1974: 1, 757–758
4. Benbassat J, Gefel D, Larholt K *et al.* Prognostic factors in polymyositis/dermatomyositis. A computer assisted analysis of ninety-two cases. *Arthritis Rheum.* 1985: 28, 249–255

5.1   INTRACTABLE DISEASE

History

J.H., a metallurgist, first became unwell in 1975 when he developed a febrile illness and some joint pains. A week later he found increasing difficulty in walking and rising from a sitting position, and by the following week could not even get out of a bath. He was referred to his local hospital where a diagnosis of polymyositis was made on the basis of elevated serum muscle enzymes, a typical EMG and a muscle biopsy. He was initially treated with a high dose of prednisolone, but following a relapse in 1979 azathioprine was added. He achieved a prolonged remission, lasting until 1981, when he had a further flare which only partially responded to an increase in prednisolone. Intravenous methotrexate was started (25 mg weekly, increasing to 50 mg) with little benefit. At this point he was referred to our unit for review and base-line investigations.

INVESTIGATIONS

Hb	10.1 g/dl, normochromic normocytic
WC	12.3×10^9/L
ESR	90 mm/h
AST	140 IU/L
CPK	1200 IU/L
LDH	500 IU/L
EMG	typical of myositis
Biopsy	intense inflammatory cell infiltrate with degeneration of muscle fibres
ANA	negative
ENAs	anti-Jo-1 antibody present

Progress and management

In view of his profound and increasing muscle weakness with declining ventilatory function, a trial of total body irradiation was given to a total dose of 200 cGy (rads) over a period of 10 weeks, whilst keeping his maintenance dose of prednisolone at 20 mg daily. The response was dramatic (Figure 5.1)

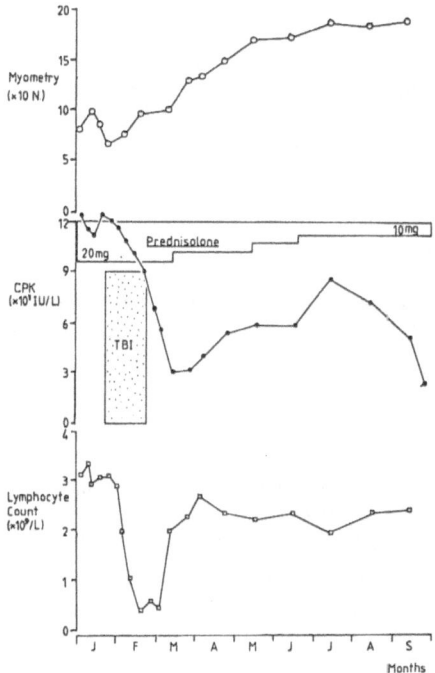

Figure 5.1 Patient's response to total body irradiation

with a fall in CPK two weeks after starting treatment concomitant with the development of a lymphopaenia, and improvement in muscle strength as finely monitored by strain gauge myometry. He left hospital a month later and returned to work. Three years later he remains well although his CPK has never returned to normal.

Points for discussion

Polymyositis may run a chronic and debilitating course with appreciable mortality. Incapacity may be permanent and death can occur from pneumonia, cardiac involvement or complications of treatment.

Following earlier successful reports of TBI in treatment of myositis and, in view of this man's declining condition, the decision to treat aggressively in this way is justified although the duration of response is unpredicatable.

Muscle destruction in myositis is thought to involve a subset of cytotoxic lymphocytes, although myositis-specific autoantibodies have been implicated. Irradiation can have diverse effects on lymphocytes, and, in all patients we have treated this way, a lymphopaenia has resulted. It should be remembered that severe marrow suppression with all its hazards can occur, especially in patients such as these, where the marrow has already been sensitized by treatment with other cytotoxic drugs.

Comment

This and other similar cases suggests that TBI might have a role in life-threatening polymyositis, if only to 'buy time' until other therapy takes effect.

References

1. Engel W K, Richter A S and Galdi A P. Polymyositis; remarkable response to total body irradiation. *Lancet* 1981: 1, 658 (letter)
2. Hubbard W N, Walport M D, Halnan K E *et al*. Remission from polymyositis after total body irradiation. *Br. Med. J.* 1982: 285, 1915–1916
3. Morgan S H, Bernstein R M, Coppen J *et al*. Total body irradiation and the course of polymyositis. *Arthritis Rheum.* 1985: 28, 831–835

5.2   A USEFUL CLINICAL 'LABEL'

History

At the age of 46 Mrs P.R. had to consult her GP when she developed a carpal tunnel syndrome. He successfully treated this with a steroid injection, but she continued to be troubled with arthralgias and developed a scaly rash over her elbows and knuckles which he diagnosed as psoriasis. The rash cleared with topical steroids, but her joint symptoms persisted although there was some response to NSAIDs, and, over the winter, she developed marked Raynaud's phenomenon.

Two years later, she was referred to her local chest clinic having complained of a dry cough and breathlessness on exertion. She had clubbing and a clinical and radiological diagnosis of fibrosing alveolitis was made, confirmed by transbronchial lung biopsy. She was given high-dose prednisolone (40 mg daily) and gradually reduced to a maintenance dose. Her joint symtoms disappeared.

A year later she was admitted to her local hospital as an emergency having developed high fevers, myalgias and a profound proximal myopathy. A diagnosis of polymyositis was made on the basis of an elevated creatinine kinase (1200 IU/L) and EMG. The prednisolone was increased to 60 mg daily and she was transferred to our unit.

Investigations

FBC	within normal limits
ESR	56 mm/h
Immunoglobulins	
RA latex test	
ANA	
DNA-binding	normal or negative
Immune complexes	
Cryoglobulins	
ENAs	positive – anti Jo-1 antibody
EMG + muscle biopsy	active myositis
Schirmer's test	dry
Labial gland biopsy	lymphocytic infiltration

CXR and lung function test compatible with fibrosing alveolitis (Figure 5.2).

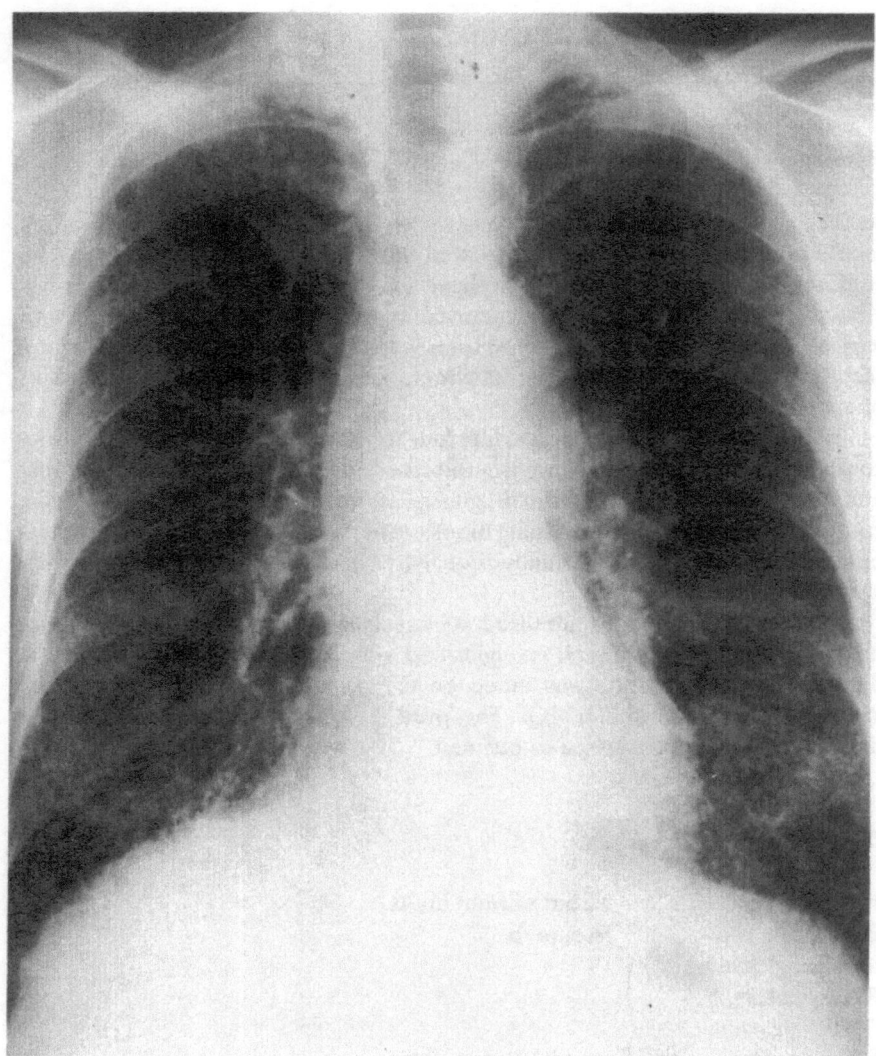

Figure 5.2 Chest X-ray showing basal fibrosis

Progress and management

Clinical improvement on prednisolone alone was incomplete as judged by serial strain gauge myometry. There was further improvement on azathio-

126

prine but addition of this drug did not prevent flares of disease activity on reduction of steroid dose. Methotrexate, given as weekly intravenous boluses of 50 mg, resulted in sustained remission with a fall in muscle enzymes to within normal levels. Her lung function has remained stable during several years of follow-up.

Points for discussion

Pulmonary disease is an important cause of morbidity and mortality in polymyositis – occurring in some form in 50% of patients (Table 5.2).

Pneumonias form the main group, fibrosing alveolitis occurring in 5–15% of patients. The fibrosis is pathologically indistinguishable from the so-called 'cryptogenic' fibrosing alveolitis described by Hamman and Rich in 1939. This type of interstitial lung disease may complicate a number of other autoimmune disease, including rheumatoid disease, SLE, scleroderma, Sjögren's syndrome, inflammatory bowel disease and chronic active hepatitis.

This patient had an unusual antibody–antigen system, characterized by anti-Jo-1 antibody in her serum. This antibody is one of few where the antigen has been accurately defined (histidyl tRNA synthetase) and is almost exclusively found in polymyositis, especially if complicated by fibrosing alveolitis and other mild overlap features (Sicca and Raynaud's). It is also of interest and perhaps of some clinical note that we have to date not found this antibody in patients with childhood or malignancy-associated myositis.

Clinically evident fibrosing alveolitis often, as in this case, preceeds the onset of muscle disease, and does seem to differ from the idiopathic form in its favourable response to steroids.

Table 5.2 Pulmonary complications of myositis

1. Complicating the disease

   Ventilatory insufficiency
   Aspiration pneumonitis
   Hypostatic pneumonia
   Fibrosing alveolitis (CFA)

2. Complicating treatment

   Opportunistic infection
   Drug-induced fibrosis (methotrexate)

Comment

Anti-Jo-1, of all the cytoplasmic and nuclear antibodies, appears to have considerable specificity, and therefore clinical diagnostic value, in defining the subset of patients with myositis and pulmonary fibrosis.

References

1. Dickey B F and Myers A R. Pulmonary disease in polymyositis/dermatomyositis. *Semin. Arthritis Rheum.* 1984: **14**, 60–76
2. Mathews M B and Bernstein R M. Myositis autoantibody inhibits histidyl tRNA synthetase. A model for autoimmunity. *Nature* 1983: **304**, 177–179
3. Bernstein R M, Morgan S H and Bunn O C. 1 Anti Jo-1 antibody: a marker for myositis with interstitial lung disease. *Br. Med. J.* 1984: **289**, 151–152

5.3   CONDUCTION ABNORMALITIES

History

Colin, a 41-year-old office clerk, had been well all his life until he fell and twisted his knee, developing an effusion. This settled with rest, but the muscles in both legs felt continually 'uncomfortable' despite physiotherapy.

Three months later he collapsed on his way to work. This was a true 'blackout' lasting several seconds, with no features suggestive of epilepsy. He didn't consult his GP further until several weeks later when the syncopal episodes were occurring up to 10 times/day. He had also begun to feel weak, with pain in his pectoral muscles, and some proximal weakness in both legs. His GP recorded his pulse rate at 40/min and immediately referred him to hospital.

Investigations

Hb	14 g/dl
WC	14×10^9/L neutrophilia
ESR	46 mm/h
CPK	8000 IU/L
ECG	complete heart block

Progress and management

A temporary pacemaker was inserted and subsequently replaced with a permanent wire. His other muscle enzymes (AST, LDH) were also abnormally high. An EMG suggested a diagnosis of polymyositis, and active inflammation with some necrosis was seen on a sample of muscle obtained by quadriceps needle muscle biopsy. There was partial improvement in muscle function on high-dose prednisolone. Azathioprine was added but withdrawn because of a persistently elevated GT and alkaline phosphatase. These did not subside and a liver biopsy was performed. This showed early fibrosis as well as marked fatty steatosis. On subsequent questioning, he admitted that he had underplayed his alcohol intake somewhat. This precluded the use of methotrexate and he was maintained on varying levels of prednisolone.

129

Points for discussion

Inflammatory myocardial involvement in myositis is rare but well described. Mitral valve abnormalities and conduction defects, on the other hand, are found more commonly, especially the latter. Some studies report an incidence of ECG abnormalities between 30 and 40% although these are not necessarily symptomatic. ·

Some workers have placed emphasis on the use of measuring relative levels of the CK-MB isoenzyme of creatinine kinase in detecting myocardial involvement, although we have found this to be of little value in our unit.

This patient illustrates some of the therapeutic problems in patients whose muscle disease only responds partially to steroids.

Comment

This case also highlights the difficulties seen in the treatment of polymyositis – often a disease which proves more difficult in practice than in the textbooks.

References

1. Gottdiener J S, Sherber H S and Engel W K. Cardiac manifestations in polymyositis. *Am. J. Cardiol.* 1978: **41**, 1141–1149
2. Stern R, Gobold J H, Chess Q and Kagen L J. ECG abnormalities in polymyositis. *Arch. Intern. Med.* 1984: **144**, 2185–2189
3. Strongwater S L, Anesley T and Schnitzner T J. Myocardial involvement in polymyositis. *J. Rheumatol.* 1983: **10**, 459–463

Section 6

SCLERODERMA

INTRODUCTION

Scleroderma (progressive systemic sclerosis – PSS) is a generalized disorder of connective tissue characterized by fibrosis and subsequently damaging degenerative and atrophic complications. The disease is dominated by its cutaneous manifestations which may be mimicked by a number of other pathological conditions. A broad classification of sclerodermatous conditions is shown in Table 6.0.

Table 6.0 Sclerodermatous diseases

Localized cutaneous scleroderma
      morphoea – single or multiple plaques
      linear scleroderma

Systemic sclerosis
      'CREST' syndrome
      diffuse systemic sclerosis
      'overlap' syndromes

Eosinophilic fascitis

Chemical/drug induced
      vinyl chloride
      bleomycin

Graft-versus-host disease

Lichen sclerosis et atrophicus

The aetiology is unknown, but there is, in common with many of the connective tissue diseases, a peculiar predilection for the female (male: female 1:5). The almost universal occurence of Raynaud's phenomenon, which may precede other disease manifestations, should alert clinicians to suspect the possibility of PSS in women presenting with this symptom.

The diagnosis is made on clinical grounds, and some 60% of patients may have antinuclear antibodies with a speckled, or nuclear pattern of immuno-fluorescence. More specific characterization of these antibodies demonstrates anti-Scl-70 and anti-centromere antibodies, the latter being particularly common in 'CREST' syndrome.

A variety of specific therapies have been advocated, including colchicine,

D-penicillamine and plasma exchange, but, to date, their value has not been validated by carefully controlled clinical trials.

Although, in many ways, the diagnosis of PSS would seem futile in terms of possible therapeutic options, the following clinical situations should bear careful assessment.

Oesophagitis – the use of H_2 antagonists such as cimetidine and ranitidine may dramatically provide symptomatic relief, as well as improving appetite.

Raynaud's – calcium channel blocking agents like nifedipine may reduce this painful manifestation and protect against digital gangrene.

Diarrhoea – should be carefully assessed to exclude treatable causes, including bacterial overgrowth which often responds to a short course of antibiotics.

Hypertension – which is often sudden and 'malignant' in its presentation, heralds a 'turn for the worse', often with a precipitous decline in renal function. The development of angiotensin converting enzyme (ACE) inhibitors may postpone this inevitable scenario.

Steroid therapy – should be reserved for patients whose disease is complicated by inflammatory muscle disease (myositis) or interstitial lung disease

Further reading

1. Medsger T A Jr. Progressive systemic sclerosis. *Clin. Rheum. Dis.* 1983: 9, 655–670
2. Hayes D C and Gershwin H E. Immunopathology of progressive systemic sclerosis (PSS). *Semin. Arthritis Rheum.* 1982: 11, 331–351
3. LeRoy E C. Scleroderma (systemic sclerosis). In Kelley W N, Harris E D, Ruddy S *et al.* (eds.) *Textbook of Rheumatology* 1979, Philadelphia, Lea & Febiger, pp. 762–809

6.1   RENAL FAILURE

History

Joan, aged 50 years, first presented to her general practitioner in 1980 with classical Raynaud's phenomenon. On examination, she had a 'pinched' face with tightness of the skin over her cheeks and extensive telangiectasia. Her blood pressure was high and a number of investigations were found to be abnormal.

Investigations

Hb	11.2 g/dl
ESR	89 mm/h
Urea	22 mmol/L
Creatinine	305 mcmol/L

Progress and management

She was admitted to her local hospital, where further investigation of the renal impairment was pursued. An intravenous urogram demonstrated gross dilatation of both pelvicalyceal systems and ureters (Figure 6.1). The features were compatible with retroperitoneal fibrosis, and after relief of the obstruction by temporary nephrostomies a left ureterolysis and a right uretero–ileocystoplasty were performed and extensive fibrosis confirmed. A diagnosis of the 'CREST' variant of scleroderma was made on the basis of extensive digital calcinosis and tuft resorption radiologically, and a barium swallow which was compatible with hypomotility. She was discharged on oral steroid therapy with only mild impairment of renal function.

Points for discussion

Renal failure complicating scleroderma, as is also exemplified by Case 6.2, is usually associated with a poor prognosis. The presentation may often be abrupt with hypertension, and, although careful supervision and the use of angiotensin-converting enzyme (ACE) inhibitors may prolong the time

course, end-stage renal failure usually promptly supervenes.
Interestingly, she was found to be HLA-B27 positive on tissue typing!

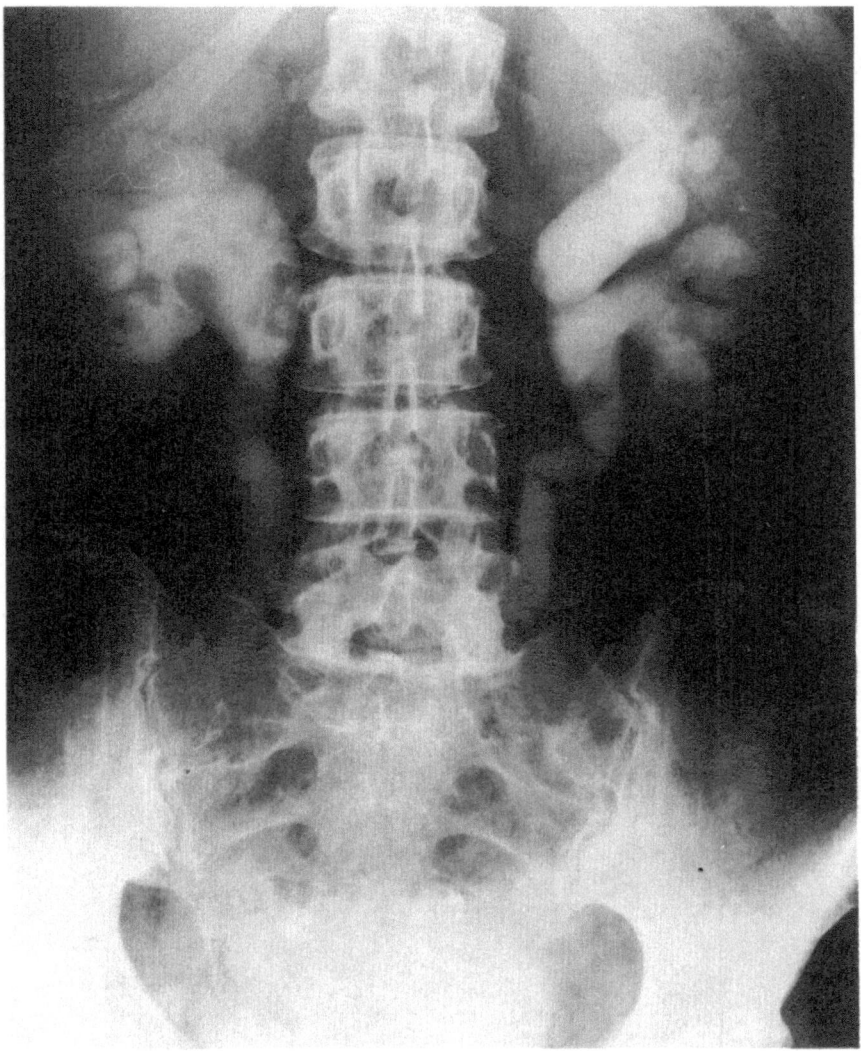

Figure 6.1 Characteristic changes of retroperitoneal fibrosis on IVU

Comment

This patient reminds us of a pertinent lesson – in many of the connective tissue diseases, other causes for renal impairment should be pursued.

References

1. Willscher M K, Novicki D E and Cwazka W F. Association of HLA-B27 antigen with retroperitoneal fibrosis. *J. Urol.* 1978: 120, 631–633
2. Rabin B S, Rednan G B, Basjian S and Gill T J. HLA antigens in progressive systemic sclerosis. *Arthritis Rheum.* 1975: 18, 381–382

6.2   FULMINANT SYSTEMIC SCLEROSIS

History

V.C., a 26-year-old Caucasian female spot welder, presented in outpatients with a four-month history of pain and stiffness in the knees, particularly in the early mornings and after immobility. She had lost weight and suffered from Raynaud's phenomenon for only a few months. Her mother had rheumatoid arthritis. When examined, she had a blood pressure of 140/80, sclerodactyly (Figure 6.2) and a mild synovitis of metacarpophalangeal joints, wrists, hips and knees. She was treated with a non-steroidal anti-inflammatory drug, and investigations were instigated.

One month later, she was admitted for a routine minor surgical procedure, but she complained of severe pain in her joints, and increasing breathlessness on exercise. In the preceding 24 hours, she had become markedly more breathless, even at rest, and had suffered episodic left-side chest pain, which was sometimes pleuritic in nature.

Examination

An unwell, pyrexial patient with sclerodactyly, a regular tachycardia, raised jugular venous pressure, gallop rhythm, blood pressure of 170/100 with no paradox, and bilateral posterior basal crackles in her chest.

Investigations

FBC	normal
ESR	13 mm/h
C-reactive protein	33 mg/L
Urea	4.3 mmol/L
Creatinine	53 mcmol/L
Creatine phosphokinase	11
Antinuclear factor	1:10 speckled immunofluorescence
DNA antibody	negative
Complement profile	normal
Chest X-ray	bilateral fine interstitial shadowing

ECG	small complexes, T wave depression in the lateral anterior chest leads
Echocardiogram	large left atrium and ventricle, mild mitral, pulmonary and tricuspid regurgitation
Ventilation/perfusion lung scan	normal
Blood gases	pH 7.47 pO_2 54 mmHg pCO_2 32 mmHg

Progress and management

Within twenty-four hours of admission, the patient became considerably more breathless and had a respiratory arrest. Her blood pressure was 230/130 mmHg. She required assisted ventilation, diuretics and an intravenous nitroprusside infusion. A revised diagnosis of systemic sclerosis of the kidneys, malignant hypertension and left ventricular failure was made. She was converted to oral antihypertensive therapy in the form of nifedipine and, later, captopril. Her renal function tests now became abnormal and steadily deteriorated. Her blood pressure became increasingly difficult to control and her cardiovascular state became unstable once more. Acute renal failure ensued, and the patient died only two months after her initial presentation.

Post-mortem findings

Skin	Hyaline sclerosis of the dermal collagen with entrapment of sweat glands
Lungs	Interstitial and pleural oedema
	Interstitial fibrosis
Kidneys	Extensive cortical infarction
	Fibrinoid change in the arcuate and interlobular arteries and arterioles; focal calcification in the medulla
Heart	Widespread foci of recent infarction
	Foci of longer-standing myocardial fibrosis
	No vascular occlusion
Summary	Extensive thrombotic microangiopathy resulting in extensive infarction of the kidney, heart and colon, with skin changes of scleroderma

Points for discussion

We failed. This patient demonstrates the worst end of the spectrum of scleroderma and the remarkable rapidity with which it can inexorably progress, with the clinician unable to arrest it.

In systemic sclerosis, 80% of patients closely studied are said to have at least subclinical disease of the heart. Pericardial disease is generally prominent, arrhythmias and sudden death occur, but congestive cardiac failure is uncommon. Although nifedipine has been reported as potentially helpful in disease of the heart, treatment is essentially symptomatic. It is important to note that malignant hypertension usually occurs where there is prominent skin and other visceral involvement, but may occur with devastating rapidity. Despite reports of successful treatment of malignant hypertension in systemic sclerosis, a successful outcome would seem to be the exception, rather than the rule, and the renal disease generally progresses. The major features of renal disease in systemic sclerosis are proteinuria (1/3rd), hypertension (1/4th), uraemia (1/5th), with malignant hypertension only occurring in 7%. Renal involvement has an enormous effect on the progress of patients with systemic sclerosis, with the mean time of death after appearance of the hypertension being thirteen months, after proteinuria being seven months, and after malignant hypertension being one month only.

Comment

This complication of scleroderma – reno-vascular hypertension – still defies adequate treatment.

References

1. Clements P J, Furst D E and Cabeen W *et al.* The relationship of arrhythmias and conduction disturbances to other manifestations of cardiopulmonary disease in progressive systemic sclerosis. *Am. J. Med.* 1981: **71**, 38 – 46
2. Bulbley B H, Rudolf RL, Salyer W R *et al.* Myocardial lesions of progressive systemic sclerosis. A cause of cardiac dysfunction. *Circulation* 1976: **53**, 483 – 490
3. Wasner C, Coobe C R and Fres J F. Successful medical treatment of scleroderma renal crisis. *N. Engl. J. Med.* 1978: **299**, 873 – 875
4. Traub Y M, Shapiro A P, Rodnan G P *et al.* Hypertension and renal failure (scleroderma renal crisis) in progressive systemic sclerosis. Review of a twenty – five year experience with sixty-eight cases. *Medicine (Baltimore)* 1983: **62**, 335 – 352
5. Cannon P J, Hassar M, Case D B *et al.* The relationship of hypertension and renal failure in scleroderma to structural and functional abnormalities of the renal cortical circulation. *Medicine (Baltimore)* 1974: **53**, 1 – 46

6.3   GRAFT-VERSUS-HOST DISEASE

History

A 25-year-old white male with aplastic anaemia had a bone marrow transplant from an unrelated donor in 1982. Post-graft immunosuppression was, as usual, although cyclosporin had to be avoided in view of a previous hypersensitivity reaction.

Post-transplantation, he developed recurrent oropharyngeal herpes, and within a few months his skin had become 'sclerodermatous' (Figure 6.3). He had noted persistent grittiness of the eyes.

The next two years were complicated by numerous infections, and chronic diarrhoea. The skin overlying his chest became ulcerated and he was severely incapacitated by flexion contractures of both elbows. There was marked scarring alopecia, and he complained of muscle weakness.

Progress and management

Cyclosporin was reintroduced, but again resulted in a hypersensitivity reaction. A trial of penicillamine was ineffective and his general condition deteriorated. Following a long period of being completely housebound, he died.

Points for discussion

This patient displayed chronic graft-versus-host disease (GVHD) in its most prolific form. GVHD is precipitated by the response of donor T lymphocytes in the marrow graft to antigens expressed on host cells. The clinical 'expression' is due to cytotoxic effector mechanisms and production and recruitment of monocytes by lymphokines.

GVHD may be acute or as in this patient chronic. Acute GVHD is common, occuring in 50–70% of patients and 1/3 of these patients succumb. Chronic GVHD is more unusual (15–40%). The clinical features are listed:

*   Generalized cutaneous eruptions
*   Widespread sclerodermatous changes
*   Joint contractures

140

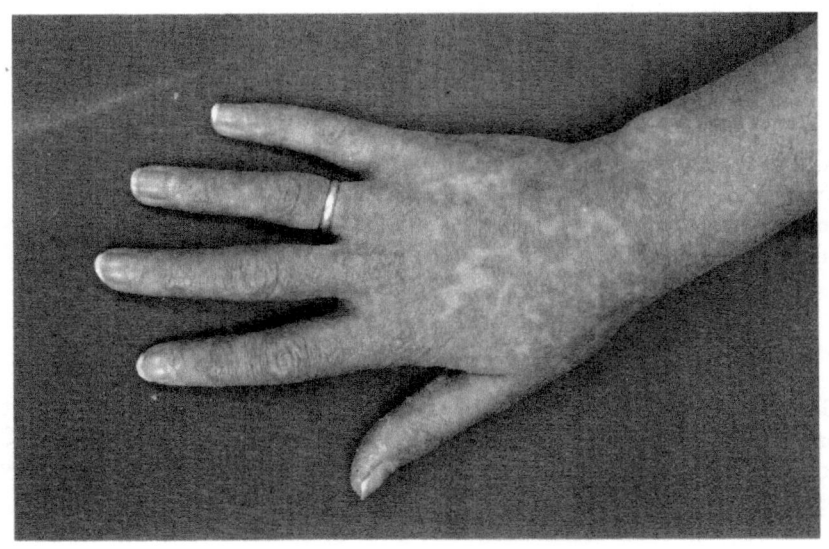

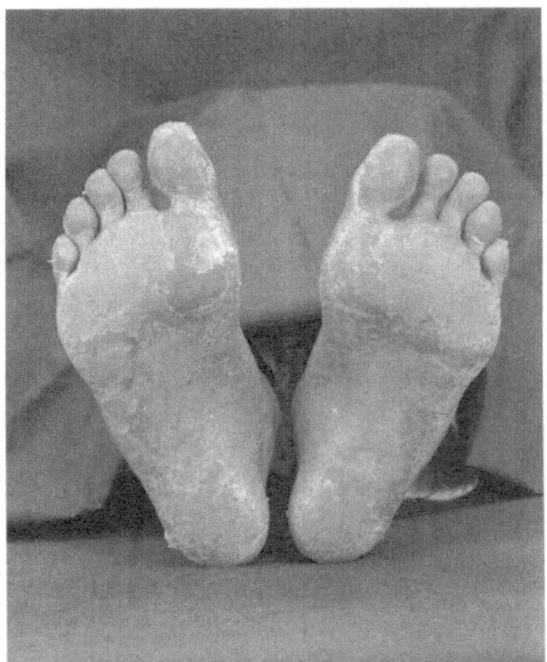

Figure 6.3 Skin changes in graft-versus-host disease

* Sicca syndrome
* Malabsorption
* Biliary cirrhosis
* Severe immunosuppression

A number of treatments have been used with varying degrees of success. Cyclosporin A, which specifically inhibits activation of T cells triggered by antigen, has greatly improved survival in marrow transplantation, as well as in other forms of organ transplantation.

Comment

Graft-versus-host disease has become a 'catch-all' in discussions of the pathogenesis of certain autoimmune diseases. Although the skin lesions differ somewhat from scleroderma, the lessons gained by the analogies *have* proved useful.

References

1. Barrett A J and Gordon-Smith E C. *Bone Marrow Transplantation, A Review.* 1983 (Oxford Medicine Publishing Foundation)
2. Denman A H. Graft versus host diseases: new versions of old problems. *Br. Med. J.* 1985: **290**, 658–660
3. Harper J I. Cutaneous graft versus host disease. *Br. Med. J.* 1987: **295**, 401–402
4. Deeg H J, Storb R and Thomas E D. Bone marrow transplantation. A review of delayed complications. *Br. J. Haematol.* 1984: **57**, 185–208
5. Graham-Brown R A C and Sarkany I. Scleroderma-like changes due to chronic graft-versus-host disease. *Clin. Exp. Dermatol.* 1983: **8**, 531–538

6.4   ATHLETE'S FOOT

History

An amateur boxer in his late 20s noticed increasing tenderness in the muscles of both forearms and calves with some redness of the overlying skin. This followed a period during which he had been training rigorously. Over the ensuing weeks the skin of his forearms and around the ankles became more inflamed and indurated and he sought medical advice.

Progress and management

On examination he had thickening of the skin of his hands and forearms. This was also present around the ankles, where the distribution accurately followed the line of his boxing boots (Figure 6.4). There was limitation of movement in both ankles and early contractures in both elbows.

A full history did not elicit any systemic symptoms, and he had no Raynaud's or sicca features. A large number of investigations including muscle enzymes were normal except for a peripheral eosinophilia. A skin biopsy confirmed a diagnosis of eosinophilic fasciitis. The epidermis was normal, but in the dermis there was proliferation of collagen and other connective tissue with eosinophilic infiltration. There was marked oedema of the subcutis. There was a good response to oral steroids with resolution of the eosinophilia and disappearance of any further skin inflammation although the indurated areas persist.

Points for discussion

Eosinophilic fasciitis is an unusual variant of scleroderma which was first described by Shulman. In some patients it is precipitated by unusual exertion. Dermatomyositis may present similarly in its early stages, usually accompanied by Raynaud's phenomenon, sicca syndrome and dysphagia, and should be positively excluded. In most patients, a peripheral blood eosinophilia is seen, and occasionally hypergammaglobulinaemia. Moderate elevations of CPK are observed in some patients.

A rapid response to steroids is usual.

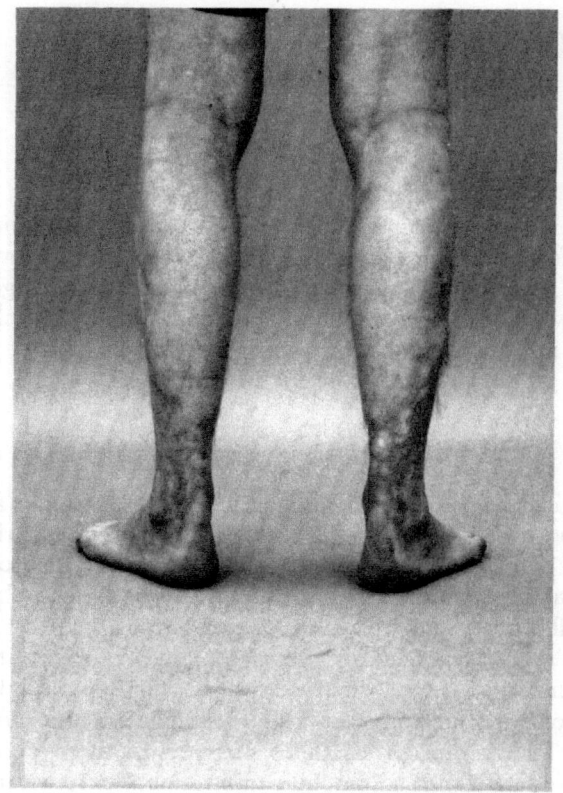

Figure 6.4 Eosinophilic fasciitis

Comment

The occasional association of this condition with haematological disease and aplastic anaemia make this syndrome less than totally benign.

Further reading

1. Shulman L E. Diffuse fasciitis with eosinophilia: A new syndrome. *Arthritis Rheum. (Suppl.)* 1977: **20**, 5205–5215
2. Moore T L and Zuckner J. Eosinophilic fasciitis. *Semin. Arthritis Rheum.* 1980: **9**, 228–235
3. Medsger T A Jr. Systemic sclerosis (scleroderma), eosinophilic fasciitis and calcinosis. In McCarty D J (ed.) *Arthritis and Allied Conditions*, 10th Edn. 1985, Philadelphia, Lea & Febiger, pp. 994–1036

6.5   OVERLAP SYNDROME

History

L.D., a 40-year-old woman, had been well until 1982 when she developed polyarthralgias and dysphagia. During that winter she had classical Raynaud's phenomenon with extreme tenderness of the nail beds. In the summer she became more unwell with chronic diarrhoea and found climbing stairs difficult. She had also noticed some difficulty breathing on exertion.

Examination

The skin over her knuckles was broken and red, and there was noticeable tightness of the facial skin with extensive telangiectasia. She was hypertensive, and had fine crackles at both lung bases. There was clinical evidence of a proximal myopathy.

Investigations

Hb	9.4 g/dl. hypochromic microcytic
ESR	44 mm/h
Folic acid studies	folate deficient
B_{12} studies	normal
Urea	12 mm/L
Creatinine	280 mcmol/L
Clearance	40 ml/min
Liver function	normal except raised AST
Muscle enzymes	all elevated
Hypergammaglobulinaemia	
RA latex test	positive 1:80
ANA	positive 1:2500 (speckled pattern)
DNA binding	normal
ENAs	positive (Pm-ScL)
Complement profile	normal
Assays for cryoglobulins and immune complexes	negative
CXR	pulmonary fibrosis

X-ray hands	digital calcinosis
Barium swallow	delayed peristalsis
Muscle biopsy	active inflammatory myositis
Labial biopsy	Sjögren's. Lymphocytic infiltrate

The clinical features and investigations were compatible with a scleroderma – myositis overlap accompanied by the presence of a characteristic antibody detected by counterimmunoelectropheresis – anti-Pm-ScL.

The myositis responded symptomatically and biochemically to high-dose steroids, but the diarrhoea persisted. A small bowel enema showed sclerodermatous involvement, but a ^{14}C breath test suggested 'stagnant' loop syndrome. Jejunal aspirates confirmed this diagnosis and the diarrhoea resolved following a course of tetracycline.

Dysphagia and control of her hypertension continue to be a problem.

Points for discussion

Rigid diagnostic demarcation of many of the multisystem diseases seen in our clinics is often not possible, features of more than one connective tissue disease often being present, as in this patient. Given time, such overlap syndromes usually delineate, with features of a more specific disease, in this case scleroderma.

The gastrointestinal tract is the most common visceral organ system to be involved in scleroderma, oesophageal disease being present in 40% of patients. It is also common in many of the scleroderma variants. Symptoms are usually due to hypomotility in the rest of the GI tract, and sclerodermatous involvement of the small bowel may produce malabsorption and intractable diarrhoea. One must however remember that bacterial overgrowth of hypomotile loops of small bowel is frequent and may cause malabsorption/diarrhoea.

A number of different autoantibodies may be found in patients with systemic sclerosis (see Table 6.5), including anti-Pm-Scl demonstrated in our patient. This was originally designated PM-1, but after multi-centre clinical evaluations it was found in a high frequency in patients with polymyositis *and* scleroderma and was renamed.

Table 6.5 Significance of ANA patterns in systemic sclerosis*

IFF staining pattern	Antigen specificity	Frequency (%)
Fine speckles	RNP	20
Fine speckles with or without nucleolar	Scl-70	10 – 30
Discrete speckles	Centromere	15 – 30
		60 – 95**
Large speckles	Unknown (matrix, midbody antigens)	10
Nucleolar (several patterns)	4 – 6S nucleolar RNA, polymerase I, fibrillarin, nucleolar organizer	60 – 70

*IFF = indirect immunofluorescence, RNA = ribonucleic acid, RNP = ribonucleoprotein, Scl = scleroderma
**Frequency for the CREST variant of scleroderma

Comment

This author is a 'splitter'. Overlap syndrome, although clinically an 'honest' label, is too easy a diagnostic dustbin. The strides made in recent years in clinical recognition of disease subsets, such as anti-Ro/SCLE, anti-Jo-1, myositis, pulmonary fibrosis, and anti-phospholipid antibodies/thrombosis, have been considerable.

References

1. D'Angelo W A. Progressive systemic sclerosis: management. 1. Introduction and general commentary. *Clin. Rheum. Dis.* 1979: 5, 263 – 276
2. Winkelmann R K. Classification and pathogenesis of scleroderma. *Mayo Clin. Proc.* 1971: 46, 83 – 91
3. Rocco V K and Hurd E R. Scleroderma and scleroderma-like disorders. *Semin. Arthritis Rheum.* 1986: 16, 22 – 69
4. Reichlin Y, Maddison P S, Targoff I *et al.* Antibodies to a nuclear/nucleolar antigen in patients with polymyositis overlap syndromes. *J. Clin. Immunol.* 1984: 4, 40 – 44

Section 7

SERONEGATIVE DISEASE

INTRODUCTION

Seronegative spondylarthropathies (SNSAs)

The 'seronegative' spondylarthropathies, although originally regarded as variants of rheumatoid arthritis, are a group of inflammatory polyarthritides in which rheumatoid factor – an IgM immunoglobulin directed against peptide determinants on the Fc fragment of human IgG, is absent. This group of diseases is nosologically distinct and separate from rheumatoid arthritis, which may also be 'seronegative', as well as other cases of arthritis.

This group comprises several different diseases:

1. Ankylosing spondylitis
2. Reiter's syndrome
3. Psoriatic arthropathy
4. 'Enteric' arthritis, associated with ulcerative colitis, Crohn's disease, by-pass surgery, Whipple's disease
5. 'Reactive' arthritis, accompanying or following bacterial/viral infections, e.g. streptococcal, *Salmonella, Shigella flexneri, Yersinia, Campylobacter, Chlamydia trachomatis*

Behçet's syndrome and adult 'Stills' disease are included by some in this category, but, strictly speaking, they do not usually demonstrate sacroiliitis and should only be included in the differential diagnosis of these conditions.

The seronegative spondylarthritides in particular share certain common features:

– Negative tests for IgM rheumatoid factor
– High frequency of sacroiliitis with or without spine involvement
– HLA-B27 antigen commonly associated
– Absence of rheumatoid nodules
– Predominantly asymmetrical, large joint arthropathy involving particularly lower limb joints
– Mucocutaneous, genital, ocular and gastrointestinal lesions are common extra articular manifestations
– 'Enthesopathy' affecting particularly tendon or ligamentous insertions into bone
– Sexually transmitted/enterically-acquired infections important in pathogenesis

- Familial 'clustering'
- Non-erosive arthropathy usually (exception: psoriatic arthropathy)

It is important to exclude other causes of 'seronegative' arthritis in younger groups and these conditions include:

- Sarcoidosis
- SLE
- Hepatitis B viraemia
- Immune complex disorders e.g. cryoglobulinaemia, Henoch–Schonlein purpura, SBE
- Adult onset Still's disease
- Behçet's syndrome
- Haemoglobinopathies

In older patients, polymyalgia rheumatica and crystal deposition disease should be considered.

'Reactive' arthritis is a term proposed as a designation for an aseptic arthritis which follows soon after an infection elsewhere and some authorities further distinguish between 'post-infectious' and 'reactive' arthritis. Assuming increasing importance in this latter type today are the arthritides following venereal or enteric infections, whereas a decade or two ago, rheumatic fever was the commonest example.

The frequency of the HLA-B27 allele in these diseases is as follows:

Ankylosing spondylitis	80–100%
Reiter's disease	60–85%
Psoriatic arthritis	20–50%
Reactive arthritis (Salmonella, Yersinia)	50–75%

In patients with psoriasis there also appears to be an increased frequency of HLA-B39, HLA-DR4, HLA-DR7, as well as a raised frequency of CW6 if a rash is present. Erosions in patients with psoriatic arthritis are associated with DR3.

The role of B27 in the pathogenesis of susceptibility is unclear and it has been suggested that B27 competes in 'molecular mimicry', the B27 antigens having antigens similar to viral or bacterial antigens. This is known as the 'cross tolerance' hypothesis.

The non-steroidal anti-inflammatory drugs (NSAIDs) are the mainstay of treatment in patients with the SNSAs, but methotrexate has recently been found to be of value, particularly in patients with resistant Reiter's syndrome.

Sulphasalazine, resuscitated as a '2nd line' therapy for the treatment of RA patients, has also proved of value in selected patients.

Further reading

1. Hasi A T and Fergesbaum S L. Seronegative rheumatoid arthritis. Fact or fiction? *Arch. Intern. Med.* 1983: **143**, 2167–2172
2. Brewerton D A. HLA B27 and the inheritance of susceptibility to rheumatic diseases. *Arthritis Rheum.* 1976: **19**, 656–668
3. Alarcon G S, Koopman W J, Acton R T *et al.* Seronegative rheumatoid arthritis: A distinct immunogenetic disease? *Arthritis Rheum.* 1982: **25**, 502–507
4. Edmonds J. Reactive arthritis. *Aust. NZ J. Med.* 1984: **14**, 81–88
5. Moll J M H. Seronegative arthropathies (Editorial). *J. Roy. Soc. Med.* 1983: **76**, 445–457
6. Ebringer A and Shipley M. Pathogenesis of HLA B27-associated diseases. *Br. J. Rheumatol.* 1983: **2**, 53–66 (Suppl.)
7. Bourne J T, Kumal P, Huskisson E C *et al.* Arthritis and coeliac disease. *Ann. Rheum. Dis.* 1985: **44**, 592–598

7.1   GOLFING HANDICAP

History

In 1980, at the age of 44, Mr R.E., manager of a local dairy, began to have a problem with his golf. This was not due to poor technique alone, as he found himself developing pain in both calves after walking only 200 yards. A referral was made to the vascular surgeons, and, after a series of investigations, the cause of this claudication was found to be due to an area of marked stenosis in the distal 3 cm of the aorta at translumbar aortography (Figure 7.1). He had surprisingly few atherogenic risk factors, being a non-smoker with normal glucose tolerance and blood lipids. He was normotensive and had a normal electrocardiogram.

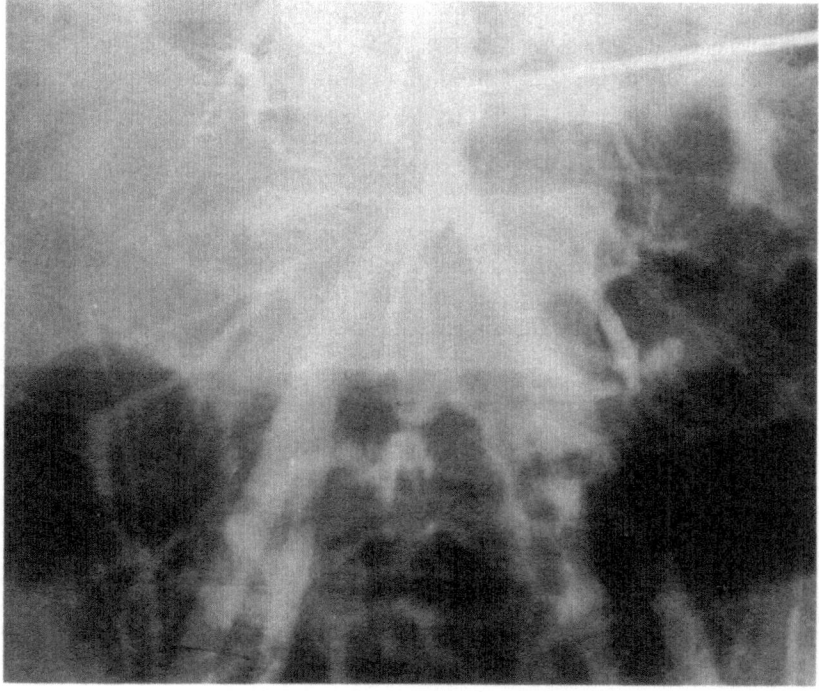

Figure 7.1 Translumbar aortogram showing distal aortal narrowing proximal to bifurcation

Progress and management

He underwent an aortoiliac bypass graft, at which minimal atheroma was found. There was extensive fibrosis and some regional lymphadenopathy, and histological examination confirmed an underlying aortitis.

The postoperative course was uncomplicated, but two years later he was referred for rheumatological advice because of severe metatarsalgia, again interfering with his golf. This had been present, only less severe, since 1978. Probing into his past history, he had had intermittent painful swelling of knees and ankles as well as low back pain. His eyes had been gritty in the mornings, and he had often sought the advice of his GP for an irritating balanitis and a rash on his feet, typical of keratoderma blenorrhagicum. The rash was originally attributed to fungal infection from his local swimming pool. He frequently had mouth ulcers. There was no other dermatological or bowel history and he had never had clinical urethritis.

An isotopic bone scan (technetium-99m) confirmed active synovitis, although there was no radiographic evidence of joint destruction. Apart from a rapid ESR (60 mm/h), all other investigations were normal. Initially he made a good response to NSAIDs, but after 6 months his symptoms could not be controlled. He was started on oral methotrexate (7.5 mg weekly) and after two months entered a remission which has lasted to date (see Case 1.5).

Points for discussion

The classical syndrome of conjunctivitis, urethritis and synovitis was described by Reiter in Prussian soldiers during the Great War of 1914–1918. Almost simultaneously, Fiessinger noted a similar illness in soldiers serving in the Somme Battle area.

The patient clearly satisfies modern criteria for this diagnosis, and has many typical clinical features (Table 7.1).

Aortic regurgitation and ascending aortitis are well documented, occurring in 3% of patients. Distal aortic involvement is extremely unusual. Conduction abnormalities, in particular, prolongation of the PR interval, are common.

The use of methotrexate in Reiter's syndrome was described as early as 1966 and, although reports are sporadic, synovitis and mucocutaneous disease appear to respond particularly favourably.

Table 7.1 Reiter's syndrome: clinical features in 131 patients

Arthritis	100%
Urethritis	88%
Low back pain	70%
Eye disease	59%
Enthesopathy	58%
Balanitis	45%
Stomatitis	25%
Keratoderma	20%
Diarrhoea	15%
Cardiovascular	10%
CNS	10%

Comment

The presence of conduction abnormalities in reactive arthritis may be a worrying aspect of the disease. Fortunately, on present evidence, these are usually subtle and rarely lead to life-threatening arrhythmias. In this case, distal disease of the aorta was seen in the absence of more widespread aortic involvement, or aortic valve disease.

Again, methotrexate is beginning to find a place in intractable and incapacitating cases.

References

1. Wilkens R F, Arnett F C, Bitter T *et al.* Reiter's syndrome. Evaluation of preliminary criteria for definite Reiter's disease. *Bull. Rheum. Dis.* 1983: **32**, 31–34
2. Good A E. Reiter's disease, a review with special attention to cardiovascular and neurological sequelae. *Semin. Arthritis Rheum.* 1974: **3**, 233–86
3. Mullins J F, Maberry J D and Stone O J. Reiter's syndrome treated with folic acid antagonists. *Arch. Dermatol.* 1966: **94**, 335–339

7.2   AN EVENTFUL HOLIDAY

History

After a camping holiday in Scotland, a 22-year-old American girl developed watery diarrhoea as well as a temperature and some low back pain. The diarrhoea settled after a week, but 10 days later she again developed a fever and difficulty weight bearing because of a swollen, painful right ankle. She was seen in casualty and referred to gastro-enterologists because of a recurrence of the diarrhoea and some diffuse abdominal tenderness. A year earlier she had been seen in America with a rash diagnosed as erythema nodosum.

Investigations

Hb	11.6 g/dl normochromic normocytic
WC	10.2×10^9/L normal differential
ESR	107 mm/h
Joint aspirate	high neutrophil count but sterile on culture
Blood cultures	sterile
Serial stool culture and microscopy	sterile

Progress and management

An initial differential diagnosis of reactive or septic arthritis was made, and she was given aspirin and flucloxacillin with resolution of the fever, although the diarrhoea persisted. A few days later she developed tenderness over the sacroiliac joints and pain in the left ankle. Both ankles were splinted to relieve the pain. Repeated stool cultures were negative, and a number of investigations, including sigmoidoscopy, rectal biopsy, barium enema and small bowel enema, were all normal.

The seemingly coincidental appearance of both diarrhoea and arthritis was irrefutable and a search for inflammatory bowel disease pursued by performing a radioisotope scan of the bowel after injection of autologous ^{111}In-labelled leukocytes. This showed abnormal localization in the otherwise radiologically normal ileocaecal region (Figure 7.2). A few days later

156

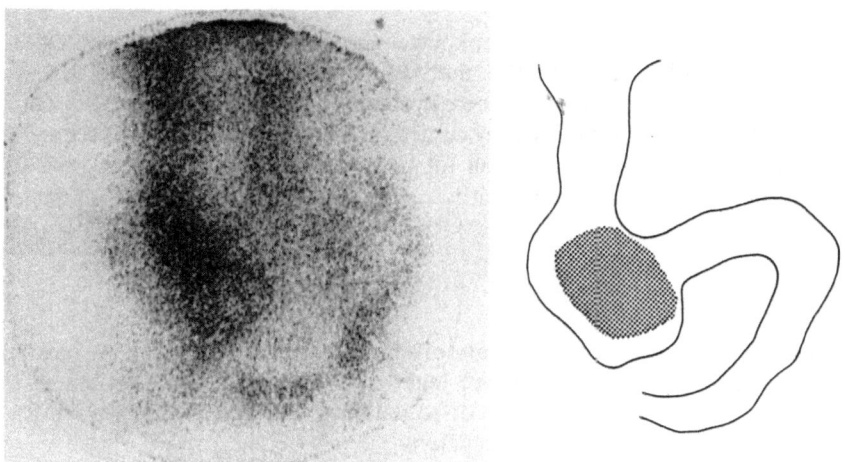

Figure 7.2 Autologous ^{111}In-labelled leukocyte scan showing abnormal localization in the ileocaecal region

agglutinins for *Yersinia enterocolitica* (serotype 0-111) were detected in the serum at a titre of 1280.

Treatment with tetracycline was started and after 3 days the diarrhoea ceased. A follow-up white cell count 5 days later was normal, and serial *Yersinia* titres fell. The arthritis symptoms settled over the ensuing month. HLA typing was A1, B8, 27 and DR3.

Points for discussion

Reactive *Yersinia* arthritis has been reported from Scandinavia and only rarely from Great Britain. As with idiopathic chronic inflammatory bowel disease, there is an acute self-limiting form, often associated with erythema nodosum and usually with diarrhoea, and a subacute or recurrent form initially triggered by infection and associated with sacroiliitis and HLA-B27. Although both forms produce predominantly lower limb arthritis with diarrhoea, the features are not sufficiently distinctive to allow diagnosis on clinical grounds alone. If stool cultures are negative, the diagnosis can be made serologically, but peak titres are not reached until the third or fourth week of illness and cannot be used at the onset. In this case, despite the prominent bowel symptoms, routine bowel radiology and histology were unhelpful.

It is established that contrast radiology may fail to detect significant bowel inflammation, and, in this case, leukocyte scanning demonstrated the lesion. Leukocyte scanning may be the method of choice for assessing disease activity in Crohn's disease and ulcerative colitis and, as in the present case, may detect inflammation missed by contrast radiography. Leukocyte scanning may also have a place in screening for underlying bowel disease in patients with seronegative or reactive arthritis.

Comment

The possibility that occult inflammatory bowel disease, negative on barium studies, might be detected by newer leukocyte scanning techniques led us to immediately screen the next dozen or so patients with acute reactive arthritis. Needless to say, the results were negative.

References

1. Ahvonen P, Seivers K and Aho K. Arthritis associated with *Yersinia enterocolitica* infection. *Acta. Rheumatol. Scand.* 1969: 15, 232–253
2. Vantrappen G, Agg H O, Ponette E, Geboes K and Bertrand P. *Yersinia enteritis* and gastroenterological aspects. *Gastroenterology* 1977: 72, 220–227
3. Elliot P R, Williams C B, Lennard-Jones J E *et al.* Colonoscopic diagnosis of minimal change colitis in patients with a normal sigmoidoscopy and normal aircontrast barium enema. *Lancet* 1983: 1, 650–651
4. Sawerymutu S H, Peters A M, Hodgson H J F *et al.* 111-Indium autologous leucocyte scanning: comparison with radiology for imaging the colon in inflammatory bowel disease. *Br. Med. J.* 1982: 285, 255–257

7.3   SURGERY FOR MORBID OBESITY

History

Mrs C.R., age 49, was first seen in our clinic in 1976 for advice regarding her unmanageable obesity. She weighed 139 kg and was 1.63 m tall. In 1978, after countless attempts at weight control, including diets, appetite suppressants, jaw wiring and self-help groups, an apronectomy and jejunoileal bypass (JIB) were performed. Three months later she had lost 38 kg in weight, but developed persistent diarrhoea and generalized arthralgias. After a year this had developed into a florid polyarthritis along with a haemorrhagic vesicular rash, mouth ulcers and febrile episodes. On admission, she was noted to have a superficial thrombophlebitis of her left leg, bilateral episcleritis and was complaining of pleuritic chest pain.

Investigations

Hb	9 g/dl macrocytic
WC	normal
Platelets	normal
ESR	60 mm/h
Vitamin B_{12}	150 mg/L
Folate	30 g/L
Iron	13 mcmol/L
Protein	63 g/L
Albumin	34 g/L
Calcium	1.98 mmol/L
Potassium	2.9 mmol/L
Liver function	normal
Immunoglobulins	normal
RA latex test	negative
ANA	negative

Immune complex and complement studies were persistently normal or negative.

Joint-radiology showed only minor degenerative changes at the knees, but a technetium-99m bone scan showed increased uptake corresponding to the clinical distribution of synovitis.

159

Progress and management

The haematological and calcium abnormalities corrected on appropriate replacement therapy, but the skin and joint problems were unremittent, despite treatment with antibiotics, NSAIDs and plasmapheresis. Dapsone reduced the frequency of exacerbations but precipitated a haemolytic anaemia.

In 1981 the bypass was reversed with full restoration of gut continuity. Her arthritis persists, and trials of colchicine, D-penicillamine and methotrexate have all failed. Her weight has steadily increased and she has had numerous readmissions for incisional hernias. She has become dependent on high doses of prednisolone to control her symptoms.

Points for discussion

JIB for morbid obesity was first introduced in 1963, and since then several complications have been recognized. These include a number of haematological and metabolic abnormalities due to malabsorption, nephrolithiasis due to to hyperoxaluria, polyarthritis, tenosynovitis, dermatitis and thrombophlebitis.

Arthritis complicates 5–30% of cases, usually symmetric and non-migratory in pattern, occurring within 3–60 months. Large joints are more frequently involved, and the disease is seronegative and non-erosive. A non-scarring vesicopapular dermatitis is often seen in association with the arthritis.

There is much controversy as to the underlying cause of these features. An abnormal immune response to intestinal bacterial antigens, absorbed from the contaminated loop has been implicated and, in the few patients where immune complexes have been isolated, such antigens have been found.

Treatment has met with variable success and efforts to suppress bacterial overgrowth using antibiotics is sometimes of value. If symptoms are severe and cannot be controlled, reversal of the JIB almost always leads to remission. Sadly, this was not the case in our patient.

Comment

Bowel disease and joint disease are often inextricably linked. Never more so than in this now-unpopular gut reversal procedure for obesity. Yet, in this patient (whose family also suffered similar syndromes of obesity, surgical bowel by-pass and arthritis) the disease was not reversed after surgery – an example of a potentially reversible arthritis becoming apparently self-perpetuating.

Obviously the popularity of this operation, quite properly, is waning. With its disappearance will also go an opportunity to study bowel disease, flora and arthritis. Nevertheless, the lessons we learnt from these patients were many – we have watched the progression, in previously arthritis-free individuals, from tenosynovitis, through a 'reactive'-pattern arthritis, to leg ulcers ('pyoderma') and finally even to features resembling Behçet's syndrome.

References

1. Leff R D, Aldo-Benson M A and Madua J A. The effect of reversion of the intestinal bypass on post-intestinal bypass arthritis. *Arthritis Rheum.* 1983: 26, 678–681
2. Zapanta M, Aldo-Benson M A, Iegel A and Madura J A. Arthritis associated with jejunoileal bypass. *Arthritis Rheum.* 1979: 22, 711–717
3. Fagan E A, Elkon K B, Griffin G F, Kennedy C, Blenkharn J J, Chadwick V S, Hughes G R V and Hodgson H J F. Systemic inflammatory complications following jejunoileal by pass. *Q. J. Med.* 1982: 204, 455–460
4. Stein H B, Schlappner O L A, Boyki W R H and Reeve C E. The intestinal bypass arthritis – dermatitis syndrome. *Arthritis Rheum.* 1981: 24, 684–690

7.4 A PAINFUL KNEE – BUT NOT ARTHRITIS

History

A 30-year-old nurse was referred to the Rheumatology Unit with painful swelling of both knees, the left more than the right. This had persisted for 3 months.

She was taking azathioprine to control Crohn's disease diagnosed 10 years earlier, and, during the investigation of her diarrhoea, a radiological diagnosis of osteopetrosis was made on the basis of characteristic end plate sclerosis in her spine (Figure 7.4). On examination she had a number of skin nodules and cafe au lait patches. There was swelling and increased warmth from the left tibial tuberosity to mid shin, but no clinical evidence of synovitis. Her brother also had the combination of Crohn's and osteopetrosis.

Investigations

Hb	13.6 g/dl macrocytic
ESR	30 mm/h
Alkaline phosphatase	175 IU/L
Acid phosphatase	10.7 IU/L
Ca^{2+} and PO_4	normal

Progress and management

The initial reason for referral had been to exclude a seronegative type of arthritis, as often complicates inflammatory bowel disease – although clinically this was clearly not the diagnosis.

The macrocytosis was attributed to azathioprine since her B_{12} and folate studies were normal. A biopsy of one of the skin nodules demonstrated histological changes of neurofibromatosis; a thorough neurological examination was normal. Radiology of the lumbar spine and pelvis confirmed the diagnosis of osteopetrosis. A 99m-methylene disphosphonate scan showed increased uptake throughout the skeleton, but was particularly marked in the area which was causing her problems. This corresponded to a lucent area on the plain X-ray of the upper tibia and fibula. An open biopsy of this area revealed histological changes that were typical of Paget's compatible with the elevated alkaline phosphatase.

162

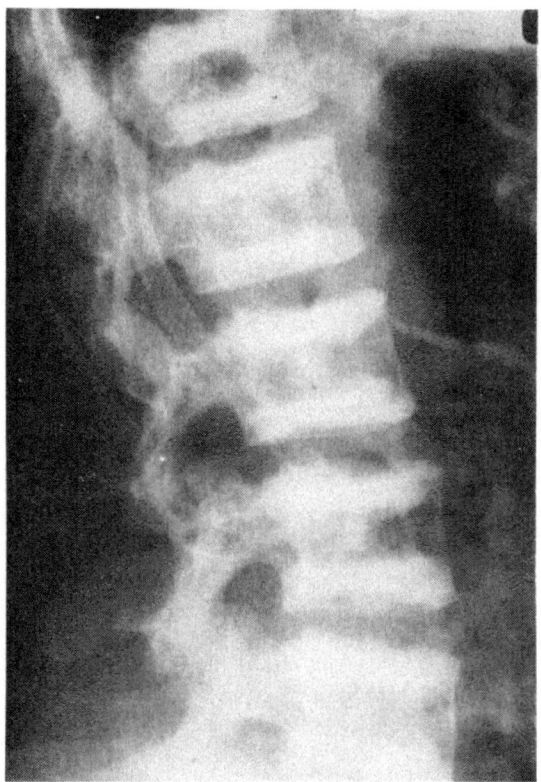

Figure 7.4 Lateral X-ray of lumbar spine showing typical 'Rugger jersey' appearance produced by sclerosis of vertebral end plates

Points for discussion

This girl was a veritable 'textbook' of unusual conditions: osteopetrosis, neurofibromatosis, Crohn's and Paget's – the latter causing her symptoms.

Osteopetrosis (Albers – Schoenberg disease) may be inherited as an autosomal dominant trait, as in this patient, and is usually asymptomatic. A recessive form also exists, characterized by fractures, hepatosplenomegaly, anaemia and early death. Elevated levels of alkaline phosphatase are not seen but the elevated acid phosphatase is typical.

Paget's complicating osteopetrosis had not previously been described. Paget's may present a variety of radiological appearances, although lucent areas within sclerotic bone are unusual.

163

Reference

1. Beighton P, Horan F and Hamersa H. A review of the osteopetroses. *Postgrad. Med. J.* 1977: **53**, 507 – 515

Section 8

CRYSTAL ARTHRITIS

INTRODUCTION

The concept of joint disease being caused by crystal deposition in the synovial membrane is still relatively new, despite the legend that gout has become in medicine and history. To date at least five types of crystalline deposits have been associated with joint disease:

*   Monosodium urate (gouty arthritis)
*   Calcium pyrophosphate dihydrate deposition disease – chondro-calcosis (CPDD) 'pseudo gout'
*   Hydroxyapatite crystal deposition disease (HADD)
*   Calcium oxalate
*   Depot corticosteroids

Monosodium urate, calcium pyrophosphate dihydrate and apatite crystals may all cause either an acute arthritis of virtually any joint, although gout most often commences in the foot. Any of these can also cause chronic polyarthritis or destructive Charcot-like arthropathy such as the 'Milwaukee shoulder' where apatite crystal deposition occurs. This severely destructive arthropathy can in fact occur with all of these crystals and involve any large joints. CPDD disease may mimic RA as symmetrical MCP, wrist and knee involvement is not uncommon. Many arthropathies due to apatite are misdiagnosed as 'culture-negative' infective arthritis as the crystals may be difficult to identify.

CPDD and apatites may be seen in patients with osteoarthritis where they may contribute to the inflammatory process. Oxalate crystal arthritis has only been reported in renal failure patients and in patients on chronic dialysis, and is secondary only to apatite as a cause of arthritis in this group of patients.

Depot corticosteroids may produce clinically significant effects in about 5% of patients and the inflammation subsides as the steroid crystals dissolve.

Crystal diseases may co-exist with infection, and synovial fluid in such patients should always be cultured. CPDD can be associated with tophus-like deposits in joints but do not cause ear tophi as are seen in gout. Hyperparathydroidism is seen in 5–15% of patients with CPDD and 40% of patients with haemochromatosis will develop the condition. Rarely, classical rheumatoid may be associated, and the diagnosis should be borne in mind, particularly in patients who are rheumatoid factor negative. Synovitis in the vicinity of the flexor tendons and a chronic dorsal synovitis of the wrists is not uncommon.

The rapidly progressive type of chondrocalcinosis may cause total joint destruction within weeks or months and this type of disease is almost invariably seen in older women in their 70s. It is usually non-articular but may be pauci or polyarticular.

In this section, we look at three patients, one with 'pseudogout' and two with true gout. Both however occurred in rather unusual circumstances.

Further reading
1. Dieppe P, Calvert P. *Crystals and Joint Disease.* 1983 (Chapman and Hall, London and New York)

8.1   POST-OPERATIVE PYREXIA

History

Mr E.G., a 46-year-old businessman, was first referred to hospital in 1982 when he was found to be hypertensive. Routine screening tests were normal apart from mild biochemical renal impairment and an elevated serum calcium. A plain abdominal X-ray revealed nephrocalcinosis. An initial diagnosis of hyperparathyroidism was supported by elevated assays for immunoactive parathyroid hormone. A [^{99}Tc]pertechnate scan suggested a parathyroid adenoma in the lower part of the left lobe of the thyroid, and this was removed at neck exploration.

Apart from a transient episode of tetany, his immediate post-operative course was uncomplicated, but after seven days he developed a high fever and a polyarthritis affecting both knees, ankles and to a lesser extent the shoulders.

Course and management

Blood cultures were taken and the episode initially treated as a post-operative sepsis. His fever did not, however, settle on antibiotics, and the arthritis became more obvious. A rheumatological opinion was sought. Joint aspirate showed small rectangular crystals which exhibited weaker positive birefringence on polarized light microscopy, typical of calcium pyrophosphate. X-rays of both knees showed fine linear chondrocalcinosis, and, interestingly, he described less severe episodes of fever and arthritis some 10 months earlier. He responded well to intra-articular steroids and NSAIDs.

Points for discussion

A large number of clinical conditions have been associated with the presence of pyrophosphate crystals (Table 8.1).

In hyperparathyroidism, crystal deposition is proportional to the duration of the disease, and it is well known that parathyroidectomy doesn't reduce the tendency to crystal deposition and indeed may encourage it, as in this patient.

Many other factors, in any case, trigger an attack of pseudogout in a

168

predisposed individual, amongst these being surgery of any kind. This usually occurs 3–10 days post-operatively, almost universally affecting the knees.

Table 8.1 Some conditions associated with deposition of pyrophosphate crystals

1.	GENERAL	Hyperthyroidism
		Haemochromatosis
		Hypothyroidism
		Gout
		Hypomagnesaemia
		Hypophosphatasia
		Steroid therapy
2	LOCAL	Joint instability
		Previous meniscectomy
		Osteochondromatosis
		Amyloidosis

Comment

This patient, with his associated disease, is, of course, younger than the usual patient. Acute pseudo gout now ranks with infection as a major cause of monarthritis of the knee in the elderly patient.

References

1. O'Duffy J D. Clinical studies of acute pseudogout attacks. *Arthritis Rheum*. 1976: **19** (Suppl. 3), 349–352
2. Pritchard M H and Jessop J D. Chondrocalcinosis in primary hyperparathyroidism. *Ann. Rheum. Dis.* 1977: **36**, 146–151

8.2   SPASTIC GAIT

History

At 33 years of age, A.R., a man well known to the hospital, was referred to the neurologists with a difficult diagnostic problem.

Grand mal epilepsy had begun at the age of 8, although this was now controlled on phenytoin, allowing him to work as a street cleaner. At the age of 15 he developed recurrent attacks of acute gouty arthritis (Figure 8.2). It was not until the age of 25 years, however, that a diagnosis of partial deficiency of hypoxanthine – guanine phosphoribosyl transferase (HPRT) was made by analysis of skin fibroblasts and erythrocytes.

On this occasion he was referred because of increasing stiffness of the legs and inability to continue to work. On examination he had signs of long tract damage in the legs with extensor plantars and a sensory level on the right to D5. It was feared that he was developing the neurological manifestations sometimes seen with this partial enzyme deficiency but a myelogram was nonetheless performed.

Course and management

Myelography, in fact, showed a tight stenosis of the spinal canal at multiple levels between C4 and C7 by osteophytes. Following decompressive surgery, he made a significant improvement allowing his return to work. Sadly, high doses of allopurinol have failed to control his hyperuricaemia well, and at the age of 40 he has significant renal impairment and hypertension. He has again developed increasing spasticity, and on this occasion obvious cerebellar signs (with phenytoin levels in the low therapeutic range) suggestive of a degenerative disorder of his spino-cerebellar tracts. Myelography does not show any spinal stenosis.

Points for management

The Lesch – Nyhan syndrome is an X-linked disease characterized by over-production of uric acid and a central nervous system disorder comprising mental retardation, spasticity, choreoathetosis and compulsive self-mutilation.

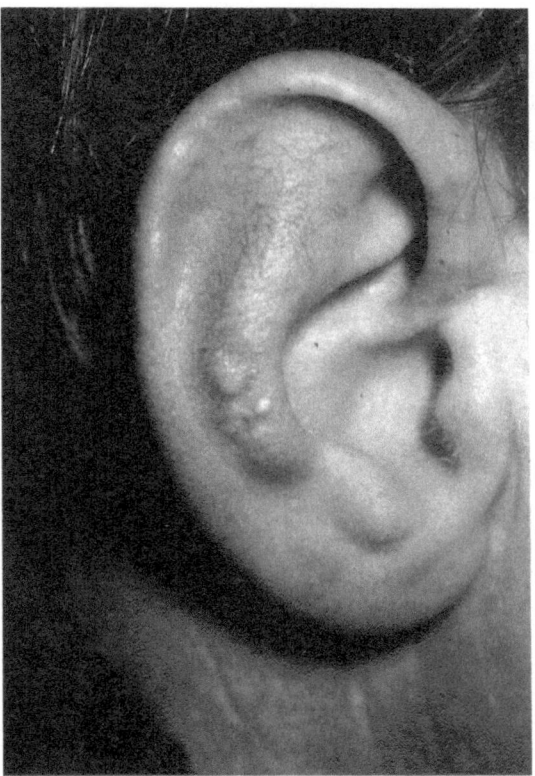

Figure 8.2 Gouty tophi

Its onset is usually at the age of 6–8 months and culminates in death due to renal failure before the age of 20 years. The underlying metabolic basis for this condition is absence of one of the enzymes involved in purine nucleotide salvage – HPRTase, although an explanation for the specificity of the neurological features remains elusive.

Many patients with partial deficiency of this enzyme have now been described. This again is X-linked, although the clinical manifestations may be variable: affected boys may be normal, or develop gout and its complications. The neurological features, if present, are less severe and life expectancy is much better.

References

1. Lesch M and Nyhan W L. A familial disorder of uric acid metabolism and central nervous system function. *Am. J. Med.* 1964: 36, 561 – 570
2. Nyhan W L. The Lesch – Nyhan syndrome. In Vinken P J and Bruyn G W. (eds.) *Handbook of Clinical Neurology* 1977: 29, 263 – 278
3. Kelley W N, Greene M L, Rosenbloom F M *et al.* Hypoxanthine – guanine phosphoribosyl-transferase deficiency in gout. *Ann. Intern. Med.* 1969: 70, 155 – 206
4. Wilson J M, Young A B and Kelley W N. Hypoxanthine – guanine phosphoribosyltransfer-ase deficiency. *N. Engl. J. Med.* 1983: 309, 900 – 910

172

8.3   ALLOPURINOL SENSITIVITY

History

Mrs M, aged 73, was found to have nodular osteoarthrosis and hypertension in 1969. Serum urate at this time was 6.8 mg/100 ml. In 1983, after a left total hip replacement for osteoarthritis, she was referred for a rheumatological opinion with symptoms of median nerve compression almost certainly due to walking stick pressure. At this time, she was found to have large tophaceous deposits in her fingers (Figure 8.3). She gave a history of several years congestive cardiac failure treated with diuretics. When subsequently admitted for median nerve decompression, her uric acid was 0.8 mmol/L, urea 4.4 mmol/L and creatinine 185 mcmol/L. Allopurinol 300 mg/day was commenced. Over the next fortnight she was unwell, with malaise, gastrointestinal upset and subsequently developed a pruritic macular rash over the trunk and limbs. Her serum urate had fallen to 0.4 mmol/L. Renal function was unchanged. Allopurinol was stopped and her rash and other symptoms resolved. A further attempt to initiate allopurinol at 100 mg/day resulted in a prompt recurrence of the rash.

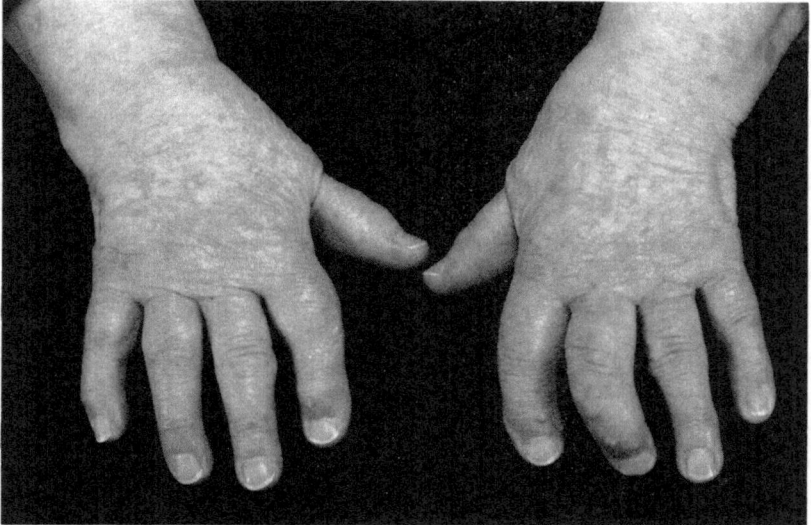

Figure 8.3 Tophaceous deposits in the hands

Progress and management

Over the next two years azapropazone and probenecid were tried without benefit. Her hyperuricaemia and tophi were aggravated by various changes to her diuretic regime. The tophi slowly enlarged and became increasingly painful.

In 1986 she was admitted for management of an infected foot ulcer aggravated by subcutaneous tophi and peripheral oedema. Investigations revealed uric acid 0.51 mmol/L, urea 18.8 mmol/L and creatinine 155 mcmol/L.

Attempts to control the oedema with increased diuretic therapy promptly increased her uric acid and caused the tophi to enlarge and ulcerate. It was decided to make a further attempt to reinstate allopurinol. This was completed without any recurrence of side effects and she was eventually maintained on 200 mg/day. On this regime her uric acid fell to 0.46 mmol/L, her tophi healed and regressed. Her renal function remained stable.

Points for discussion

This lady illustrates the classical elderly female patient with hyperuricaemia, large tophaceous deposits, but little in the way of acute gout symptoms. Such cases are a prime indication for allopurinol therapy.

As this case also shows, this situation is frequently compounded by chronic renal impairment which renders alternative hypouricaemic therapy ineffective. This situation is doubly compounded in that renal impairment may also lead to greater accummulation of the allopurinol metabolite, oxypurinol, thought to be important in mediating some of the toxic effects of allopurinol. It is possible that in this case the initial adverse reaction was in part due to the high starting dose for allopurinol and it is generally recommended that the drug is commenced in low doses, i.e. 100 mg/day in the presence of marked renal impairment. Allopurinol sensitivity may be life-threatening but is not uncommon and is a major limitation to the therapy in this particular clinical situation. Successful desensitization of patients to allopurinol preparations has been described. However, such desensitization regimes do not appear to be widely practised as judged by the sparsity of its reported usage. Such regimes deserve wider appreciation and utilization in this not uncommon situation.

References

1. MacFarlane D G and Dieppe P A. Diuretic-induced gout in elderly women. *Br. J. Rheumatol.* 1985: **24**: 155–157
2. Gibson T. Hyperuricaemic drugs. In Scott J T (ed.) *Copeman's Textbook of the Rheumatic Diseases* 6th Edn. 1986 (Churchill Livingstone) pp. 569–583
3. Ellion B, Kovensky A, Hitchins G H, Metz E and Rondalls G R W. (1966). Metabolic studies on allopurinol, an inhibitor of xanthine oxidase. *Biochem. Pharmacol.* 1966: **15**, 863–880
4. Webster E and Panush RS. Allopurinol hypersensitivity in a patient with severe, chronic, tophaceous gout. *Arthritis Rheum.* 1985: **28** (6), 707–709
5. Young J L, Boswell R B and Nies A S. Severe allopurinol hypersensitivity, association with thiazides and prior renal compromise. *Arch. Intern. Med.* 1974: **134**, 553–558
6. Meyrier A. Desensitization in a patient with chronic renal disease and severe allergy to allopurinol. *Br. Med. J.* 1976: **2**, 458
7. Kelsey S M, Struthers G R and Beswick Blake D R. Desensitization to allopurinol. *Ann. Rheum. Dis.* 1987: **46**, 84 (letter)

Section 9

MISCELLANEOUS

INTRODUCTION

Although most of the patients attending our clinics fall nicely into diagnostic 'boxes' many do not, and it is these who usually cause our sleepless nights. These patients may have a hint of this or a hint of that, but never anything definite and the investigations will be predictably normal. In offering a tertiary referral service, we also attract the unusual. We present some such cases in this section as they are a continuing source of education to us all.

9.1   A CONFUSING MIMIC

A 56-year-old West Indian van driver presented with a two-year history of recurrent swelling of the left knee. There was a moderate-sized effusion on examination, but without appreciable synovial thickening or limitation of movement. On further enquiry he complained of grittiness in both eyes and a Schirmer's test indicated much reduced tear production. There was no other joint involvement clinically but he had some patchy depigmentation of the skin over both arms and fine inspiratory crackles at both lung bases on auscultation.

Investigations

Hb	15.6 g/dl
ESR	45 mm/h
CRP	58 mg/ml
Urate	normal
IgG	24 g/L
Other immunoglobulins	normal
RA latex test	positive 1:160
ANA	negative
ENAs	negative

A Mantoux test was negative at 1:1000, the chest X-ray showed some linear collapse at both bases and, although radiographs of the knees were normal, there was some juxta-articular erosion on the metatarsal heads. Respiratory function tests were normal. Synovial fluid cultures were sterile.

Progress and management

Despite the atypical monoarticular presentation, a diagnosis of rheumatoid arthritis was thought likely in view of erosive radiographic changes, Sicca syndrome and positive tests for rheumatoid factor. There was no family history of psoriasis. There was only a partial response to NSAIDs and a synovial biopsy was performed. Surprisingly this showed villous hypertrophy and non-caseating granulomata (Figure 9.1) in keeping with sarcoidosis. A

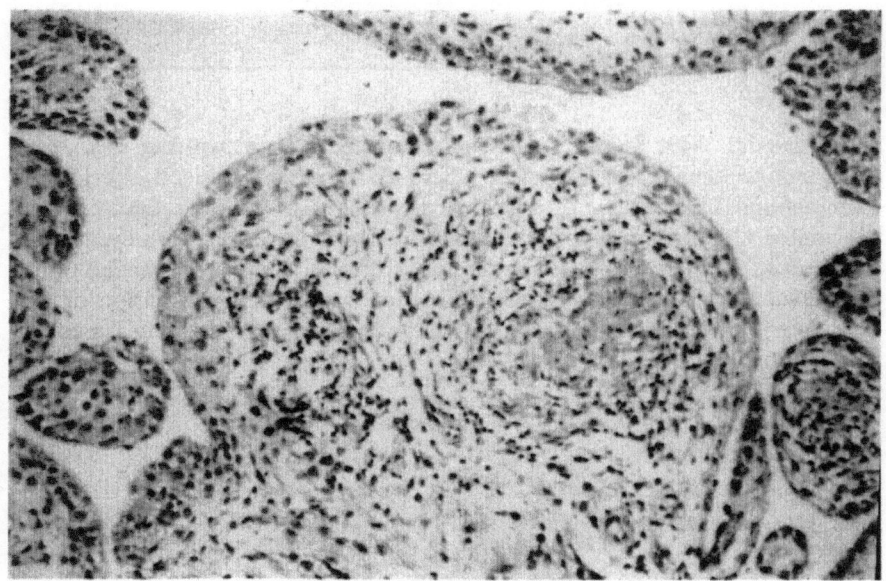

Figure 9.1 Non-caeseating granuloma in synovial biopsy

more thorough review of his past medical history through the general practitioner revealed that he had been treated for cutaneous sarcoidosis some 20 years earlier.

Points for discussion

Other than joint involvement secondary to adjacent bony disease, two types of arthritis are recognized in sarcoidosis. A non-specific, acute and transient type, occurring at the clinical onset of the disease, together with erythema nodosum, is the most common. However, a more chronic or recurrent form may occur during the later stages of the disease. This chronic granulomatous type is rare but blacks seem to be more susceptible, and, although appearing at any time during the disease course, it is generally associated with active lesions in skin and other organs.

This patient illustrates a granulomatous synovitis occurring in long-standing and apparently inactive disease, in the absence of active skin lesions or other organ involvement. The positive rheumatoid factor in this case is likely to be a function of disease chronicity, as discussed by Spilberg *et al.* A monoarthritis, the presenting feature in our patient, together with a positive rheumatoid factor, basal pulmonary fibrosis and keratoconjuctivitis sicca, contributed to the confusion in this well-known disease 'mimicker'.

Comment

A rarity – however, sarcoid and Sjögren's are not infrequent differential diagnoses in patients with joint pains, enlarged parotids, and pulmonary infiltrates. Two useful clinical pointers are the absence of positive ENA tests in sarcoid, and the potential value of a lip gland biopsy, which will not only show lymphocytic infiltrates in Sjögren's, but may also, as we discovered some years ago, show granulomota in sarcoidosis with salivary gland involvement.

References

1. Morrison J G L. Sarcoidosis in the Bantu: necrotising and mutilating forms of the disease. *Br. J. Dermatol.* 1974: **90**, 649 – 55
2. Palmer D G and Schumacher M R. Synovitis with non-specific histological changes in synovium in chronic sarcoidosis. *Ann. Rheum. Dis.* 1984; **43**, 778 – 82
3. Spilberg I, Siltzbach L E and McEwan C. The arthritis of sarcoidosis. *Arthritis Rheum.* 1969: **12**, 126 – 38

9.2   SURGICAL RISKS

History

A consultant ENT surgeon referred a 25-year-old man with Ehlers–Danlos syndrome (EDS) type 1, requesting an opinion on the patient's suitability for tonsillectomy.

The disease was first noted during early childhood with easy bruising, recurrent swelling of the knees, and dislocations. As he grew older, hyperextensibility of his skin and joint hypermobility became more evident. Following trauma, soft tissue healing was complicated by the development of a thin fragile scar, and vigorous brushing of his teeth resulted in bleeding from the gums.

Both his father and one brother also had EDS.

Progress and management

Tonsillectomy was considered appropriate because of recurrent inflammatory episodes resulting in lost time at work.

On examination, old scars were visible on forehead and knees. His skin was soft and hyperelastic (Figure 9.2), and molluscoid pseudotumours were present on the proximal forearms. All joints were hyperextensible and the 5th finger could be passively dorsiflexed to 100°. Opposition of the thumb to the flexor aspect of the wrist was achieved without difficulty. All investigations, including clotting studies and an echocardiogram to exclude mitral valve prolapse, were normal.

Points for discussion

Ehlers–Danlos syndrome is a generalized connective tissue disorder that affects skin, ligaments and tendons, as well as internal organs; it results in hyperelastic, thin, velvety and fragile skin, poor wound healing with abnormal scars, easy bruisability and joint hypermobility.

Eight types of EDS have been described, each with specific, though sometimes overlapping, features. Type 1 EDS (the gravis type) is inherited as an autosomal dominant, and is easily recognized. Skin hyperextensibility is a prominent feature, and the fold of skin which may be pulled up is often

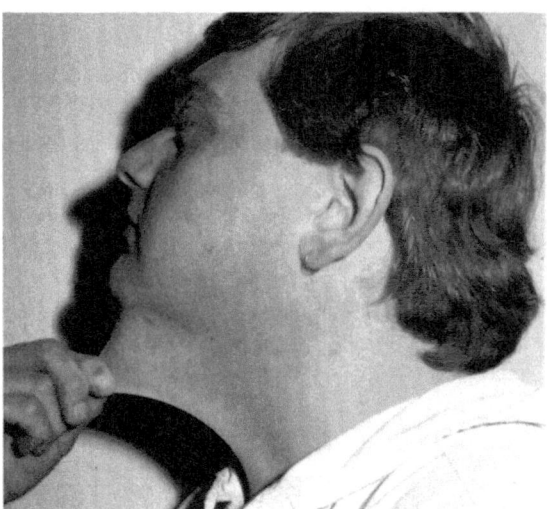

Figure 9.2 Lax skin in Ehlers–Danlos syndrome

surprisingly thin. It is velvety in appearance and feel, with a marked tendency to splitting. Easy bruising is a feature, and extremely thin 'cigarette paper' scars develop with healing following trauma. Even minor injury causes purpura or haematomas which may organize or calcify. Molluscoid pseudo-tumours and subcutaneous spheroids occur in the majority of these patients.

Prolapse of the mitral and tricuspid valves, dilatation of the aortic root or ectasia of the sinuses of Valsalva (or both), aortic valve regurgitation, and (rarely) dissecting aneurysms are among the cardiac features that have been described. In addition, various conduction abnormalities, especially right bundle branch block, have been associated with type 1 EDS.

It is in the type 1 EDS that there is a high incidence of prematurity, due to early rupture of the fetal membranes. Diaphragmatic and other hernias are fairly common and spontaneous rupture of the bowel has also been reported.

In general, the tissues in these patients are very friable, and difficulties at operation have been encountered. Bleeding may occur from tooth sockets after dental extractions, from the pharynx after tonsillectomy and at the site of joint surgery.

The patient described here has most of the cardinal features of type 1 EDS. The recommendation in cases such as these is to avoid surgery whenever possible. Prognosis, especially following a general anaesthetic, is known to be unpredictable and has been associated with intractable bleeding from the site of operation.

References

1. Vogel A, Holbrook D A, Steinmann B, Gitzelmann R and Byers P H. Abnormal collagen fibril structure in the gravis form (Type 1) of Ehlers–Danlos syndrome. *Lab. Invest.* 1979: **40**, 201–206
2. Jimenez S A and Lallay E V. Disorders of collagen structure and metabolism. *Bull. Dis.* 1979–80: **30**, 1016–1021
3. Beighton P. *The Ehlers–Danlos Syndrome.* 1970 (London: Heinemann)
4. Leier C V, Call T D, Fulkerson P K and Wooley C R. The spectrum of cardiac defects in the Ehlers–Danlos syndrome. Types 1 and 3. *Ann. Intern. Med.* 1980: **92**, 171–178

9.3   HIGH FLIERS

History

A 49-year-old military pilot presented with a painful left knee. The onset was gradual and there was no history of trauma. The joint was not swollen or hot, but extremely painful on all movements. A month later he developed pain in the left ankle, and admitted to a history of pain in the right hip ten years earlier; this was also gradual in onset and took some months to resolve. There had been no residual disability. He was generally fit but had been found to have a type 2 Friedrickson hyperlipidaemia and had a corneal arcus. There had been no evidence of ischaemic heart disease or peripheral vascular disease.

His flying career had involved piloting unpressurized aircraft to altitudes of 30 000 feet, but using oxygen.

Progress and management

Radiological examination of the left knee showed an irregular calcific mass in the epiphyseal region of the lower femur and destruction of the lateral femoral condyle. There was juxta-articular osteoporosis of both hips, with a subchondral cyst on the right and an increase in the density of the left femoral head.

A radionucleide bone scan showed increased uptake in both the left knee and ankle (Figure 9.3). The radiological changes in the knee were worryingly suggestive of chondrosarcoma and an open biopsy was performed. The histological features were described as typical of avascular necrosis, with no evidence of malignancy.

Points for discussion

Historically this man had had previous episodes of osteonecrosis, although with surprisingly little residual disability and little in the way of secondary degenerative disease, particularly in the right hip.

The causes of osteonecrosis are many (Table 9.3A) but in this man there are two important contributory factors:

185

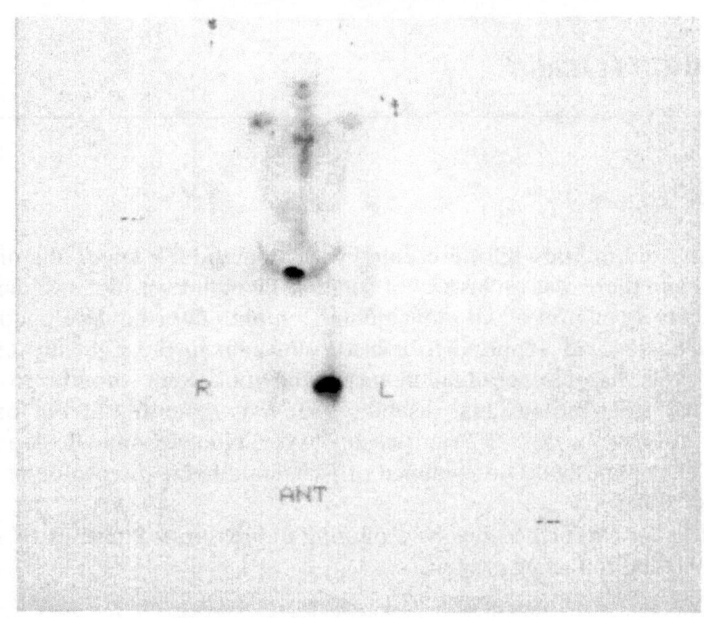

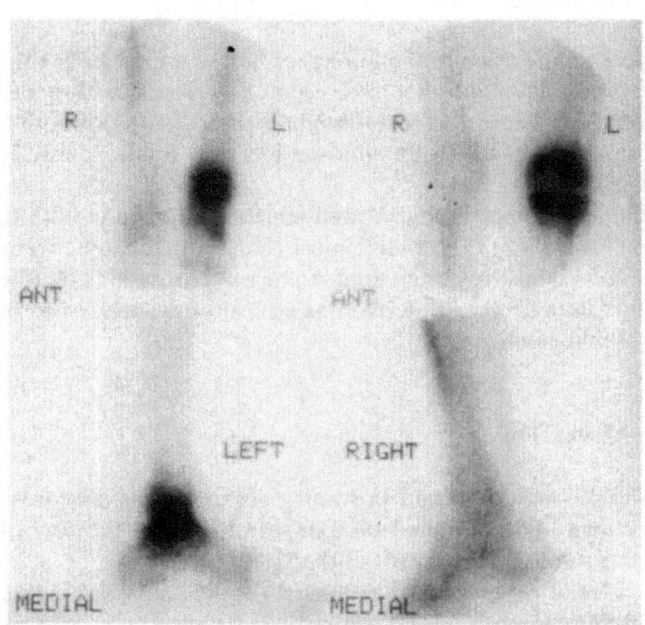

Figure 9.3 Radionucleide bone scan showing increased uptake in left knee and ankle

1. Hyperlipidaemia. Several patterns of musculoskeletal disease are associated with hyperlipidaemia (Table 9.3B). It is also suggested that hyperlipidaemia often accompanies idiopathic osteonecrosis, and may be a predisposing factor.

2. Dysbarism. This is a well known cause of osteonecrosis, and is paralleled by deep-sea divers where aseptic necrosis is more common, especially in obese and hyperlipidaemic individuals. Adipose tissue and marrow are 'slow' tissues, and supersaturation with nitrogen can occur as gas tension which may not cause obvious decompression sickness. The precise mechanism of dysbaric osteonecrosis is not clear.

Table 9.3A Causes of osteonecrosis

Trauma
Excess corticosteroids
Cushing's disease
Post renal transplant
SLE
Haemoglobinopathy
Alcoholism
Chronic liver disease
Pancreatitis
Gout
Hyperlipidaemia
Obesity
Gaucher's disease
Dysbarism

Table 9.3B Hyperlipidaemia and musculoskeletal disorders

Tendon and synovial infiltration		Mainly type II
Migratory arthritis (like rheumatic fever)		Severe in homozygous states
Polyarthritis	Episodic	Mainly types IV and V
Monoarthritis	Persistent	Often only modest
Cystic lesions		elevation of plasma lipids
Osteoporosis		
Osteonecrosis		Types II and IV
		Usually multifactorial

Scrupulous control of hyperlipidaemia results in resolution of many of the musculoskeletal manifestations, and a cholesterol-lowering agent was recommended. His future flying was restricted.

References

1. Jacobs B. Epidemiology of traumatic and non-traumatic osteonecrosis. *Clin. Orthop.* 1978: 130, 51–67
2. Chryssanthou C. Dysbaric osteonecrosis. *Clin. Orthop.* 1978: 130, 94–106
3. Buckingham R B, Bole G G and Bassett D R. Polyarthritis associated with type IV hyperlipoproteinaemia. *Arch. Intern. Med.* 1975: 135, 286–290
4. Goldman J A, Gluck C J, Abrams N R *et al.* Musculoskeletal disorders associated with type IV hyperlipoproteinaemia. *Lancet* 1972: 2, 449–452

9.4   TUBERCULOUS SYNOVITIS

History

A 26-year-old Asian woman presented to the Casualty Department with a painful right knee. Her English was limited, but there was no history of previous arthritis or psoriasis, and other joints were unaffected. She did not have a fever and was otherwise quite well. She had been in the United Kingdom for over ten years.

Except for soft tissue swelling, a plain X-ray of the knee was unremarkable and the casualty officer prescribed a course of NSAIDs. Two weeks later the patient returned complaining of more pain and increased swelling.

Progress and management

She was admitted to hospital, put on strict bed rest, and given a resting splint. The majority of investigations were normal, although the ESR was moderately elevated at 38 mm/h. Chest X-ray was normal and a joint aspiration was performed. Although the fluid was inflammatory, acid fast bacilli were not seen and there were no crystals. A Mantoux test was negative although she did not have BCG vaccination on entry to the country.

Mycobacterial infection was still suspected and an open synovial biopsy performed. The histology was compatible with tuberculosis, there being multiple granulomata, some necrotic. There was slow but definite improvement on antituberculous chemotherapy, but acid fast bacilli were never isolated from the synovium or bone biopsied.

Points for discussion

The diagnosis of a monoarthritis may often be difficult (Table 9.4), but in a patient of this racial background mycobacterial infection must obviously be excluded.

Skeletal involvement occurs but rarely in patients with tuberculosis, and a pure arthritis in the absence of local bony involvement is extremely unusual. The most frequently affected joints are the knee and hip. Occasionally tenosynovium may be involved and this can produce a carpal tunnel syndrome.

189

Active pulmonary TB is present in 20% of patients with articular disease and, once excluded, a close search for involvement of other sites must be made.

Because of the insidious nature of the disease, X-ray abnormalities are usually present by the time a diagnosis is made. Acid fast bacilli are demonstrated from synovium smears in only 20%, although 80% will be culture positive. Synovial biopsy and culture gives the best diagnostic yield. Treatment is based on conventional regimens, often starting with 4 drugs prior to obtaining sensitivities.

Table 9.4 Diagnosis of monoarthritis

Reactive arthritis
Ankylosing spondylitis
Psoriatic arthropathy
Infection
Crystal synovitis
Haemophilia
Trauma
Atypical rheumatoid

Comment

Tuberculosis synovitis, as described in this case, is rare. Tuberculosis polyarthritis (Poncet's disease) is vanishingly rare – if it ever made an appearance.

Further reading

1. Berney S, Goldstein M and Bisko R. Clinical and diagnostic features of tuberculous arthritis. *Am. J. Med.* 1972: **53**, 36 – 42
2. Goldenberg D L and Cohen A S. Arthritis due to tuberculous and fungal microorganisms. *Clin. Rheum. Dis.* 1978: **4**, 211 – 223

9.5   HYPOGAMMAGLOBULINAEMIC ARTHRITIS

History

The patient, now aged 51 years, had suffered from multiple debilitating bacterial infections since childhood, beginning at age 6 months with pneumonia. These were mainly bronchial, dental or cutaneous abcesses. Since the age of 9 she had suffered large-joint arthralgias but no objective swelling had been noted.

In December 1985 she was admitted for assessment of recurrent diarrhoea. In 1976 she had been diagnosed as having proctitis which settled spontaneously. Diarrhoea recurred in 1979 but with vomiting. Endoscopy demonstrated a benign gastric ulcer which was treated conservatively. Small bowel investigations at this time, including general biopsy, were normal. She was given sulphasalazine empirically but this led to haematological toxicity. The diarrhoea continued and she was having 5 or 6 bowel actions per day and on occasion up to 20 times a day.

Examination

Examination revealed a thin pale woman with no generalised lymphadenopathy or objective evidence of arthritis. The spleen was palpable two fingers breadth below costal margin. There were no pulmonary or neurological abnormalities detected on clinical examination.

Investigation

Hb	11.7 g/dl
WC	3.8×10^9/L (neutrophils 1.9, lymphocytes 1.7)
Platelets	161×10^9/L
ESR	3 mm/h
Serum B_{12}	661
Serum folate	7.4
Total proteins	63 g/L
Albumin	45 g/L
Globulin	18 g/L

191

Immunoglobulins:

IgG	< 0.5 g/L
IgA	< 0.1 g/L
IgM	0.1 g/L
Alkaline phosphatase	50 IU/L
Alanine aminotransferase	5 IU/L
Sigmoidoscopy	equivocally inflamed rectal mucosa
Small bowel barium meal	normal small bowel mucosa
CT scan of abdomen	normal size liver, some splenic enlargement, no significant lymphadenopathy
Stool cultures	negative (x 3)
Jejunal biopsy	normal villi, no Giardia seen
Colonoscopy	normal mucosal appearance, biopsy showed very mild inflammatory polymorphonuclear infiltrate. No crypt abscesses
Urinary senna and phenolphthalein	negative

Progress and management

Empirical treatment with metronidazole was begun but this produced only a temporary cessation of diarrhoea. Over the next six months her symptoms continued and in particular her arthralgias became increasingly severe and she lost a further 7 pounds in weight. Examination revealed marked hepato-splenomegaly and investigation showed a pancytopenia with the globulin levels unchanged. Bone marrow examination was normal. A repeat CT scan of the abdomen showed a moderate enlargement of the spleen and an enlarged retrocrural node on the right. No other lymphadenopathy was seen.

It was felt that a diagnostic laparotomy and splenectomy were needed to exclude lymphoma. At operation, a grossly enlarged spleen (923 g) was removed. The liver was noted to be enlarged and was biopsied. There were scattered small lymph nodes in the small bowel mesentery but no other abnormality.

Histology (see Figure 9.5) showed widespread infiltration of the spleen by discrete granulomata. There was focal central necrosis but no caseation and these formed confluent aggregates. All lymph nodes showed a similar appearance. The liver biopsy showed preservation of normal architecture but with scattered granulomata in the parenchyma and around portal tracts. Stains for acid fast bacilli and fungi were negative and immunohistochemistry showed a polyclonal population of T cells, B cells and plasma cells.

Post-operatively her white cell and platelet cell rose and maintained normal values at 3 month follow-up. A Kveim test was performed but was negative. A 1 in 10 000 Mantoux test was negative and the serum angiotensin converting enzyme inhibitor (ACE) was 33 (normal range 16–53). The chest X-ray was normal.

She was commenced on regular intravenous Sandoglobulin (3 g fortnightly) and long-term penicillin-V (500 mg daily). She continues to suffer arthralgias but is less troubled by infections.

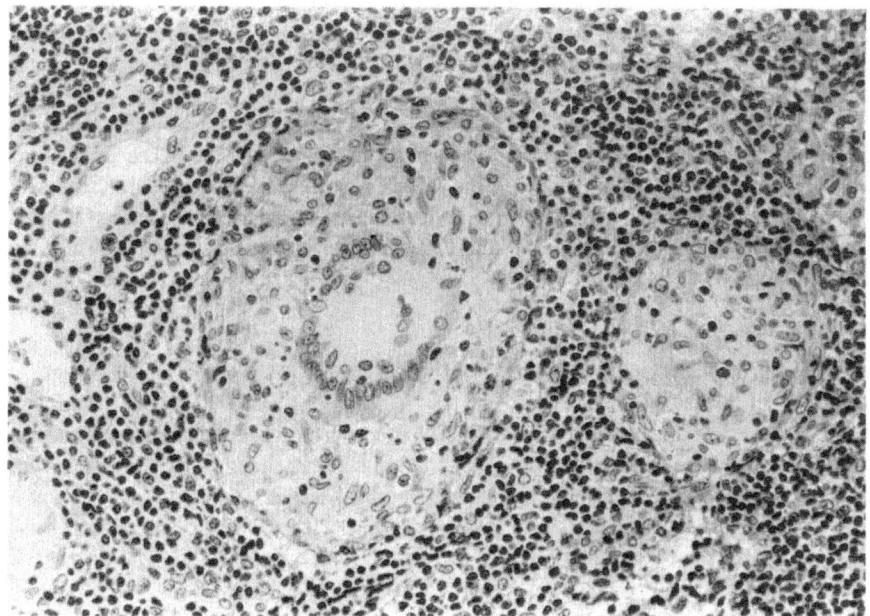

Figure 9.5 Histology of the spleen

Points for discussion

The points of interest in this case are:
1. The relationship between joint disease and immunoglobulin deficiency.
2. The occurrence of diarrhoea in the context of arthralgia and immunodeficiency.
3. The differential diagnosis of hepatosplenomegaly in immunodeficient states.

The polyarthritis associated with hypogammaglobulinaemia, although originally described as 'rheumatoid-like', has important differences. It is usually symmetrical but small joints are not so commonly involved and the arthropathy is non-erosive, non-deforming and seronegative. It frequently responds to gammaglobulin administration and our patient's poor response is unusual. It is possible that the patient had the less well-defined common variable immunodeficiency, which itself is associated with an increased incidence of autoimmune disease and malignancy, as well as chronic diarrhoea.

The classical cause of chronic diarrhoea complicating these illnesses is 'giardiasis' which may also complicate selective IgA deficiency, the commonest immunodeficiency disorder (prevalence 1 in 300 to 1 in 3000), thus reflecting the value of secretory IgA as the line of first defence against bowel pathogens.

Finally, the occurrence of sarcoid-like granulomas, although rare, is described in association with hypogammaglobulinaemia and is an important differential diagnosis from lymphoma which may also complicate this illness.

In these patients, the Kveim test is usually negative and other clinical features are absent; in particular there are no associated pulmonary abnormalities.

Comment

Years ago, the apparent association of RA with hypogammaglobulinaemia was considered an academic oddity. It seems likely that, as in this case, the chronic polyarthritis might, in fact, have been infective.

References

1. Asherson G L and Webster A D B. *Diagnosis and Treatment of Immunodeficiency Diseases.* 1980 (Oxford: Blackwell Scientific Publications)
2. Dieppe P A, Doherty M, MacFarlane D G and Maddison P J. Immunodeficiency diseases. In *Rheumatological Medicine* 1986: 11, 208 – 218 (Edinburgh: Churchill Livingstone)
3. Hansel T T, Haeney M R, Thompson R A. Primary hypogammaglobulinaemia and arthritis. *Br. Med. J.* 1987: 295, 174 – 175

9.6   CHRONIC REMUNERATIVE FIBROSITIS

The patient, a married Greek lady with two children, first complained of low backache in 1983. Myelography was complicated by a CSF leak, immobilizing her for 3 weeks with intense headaches, vomiting and dizziness. Six weeks later she underwent a laminectomy for removal of a LS/S1 disc protrusion. The low backache persisted, however, and was followed by complaints of dysplagia and vomiting. Full GI investigations did not reveal any abnormality. In January 1985 she started complaining of pain, tenderness and 'tightness' of the occipital muscles which extended over her head as well as to her sinuses, teeth and orbits. Painful 'spasms' were present over the shoulder girdle muscles and trapezii, and the pain extended paravertebrally down the spine to the sacroiliac regions on both sides. Pain was also present over both greater trochanters bilaterally. The indigestion and reflux persisted, and there were complaints of sleep problems, nightmares, tinnitus and persistently dry eyes. Nodules, often painful, appeared subperiosteally over the anterior surface of the tibiae as well as in other areas. She also complained of painful knees and ankles, sometimes accompanied by swelling. Evanescent skin lesions appeared over the lower limbs (usually purpuric and after exercise only).

Investigations

FBC	normal
ESR	1 mm/h
ANA)	
RA latex test)	negative
DNA binding)	
ENAs)	
Blood chemistry	normal
Renal and liver	
function tests	normal
Muscle enzymes	normal
Muscle biopsy	normal
Skin biopsy	questionable 'vasculitis'.
	Perivascular lymphocytic 'cuffing' only

Gastrointestinal X-rays)
Joint survey) normal
Bone scans)
Schirmer's test negative
Viral antibody titres negative
EMGs normal

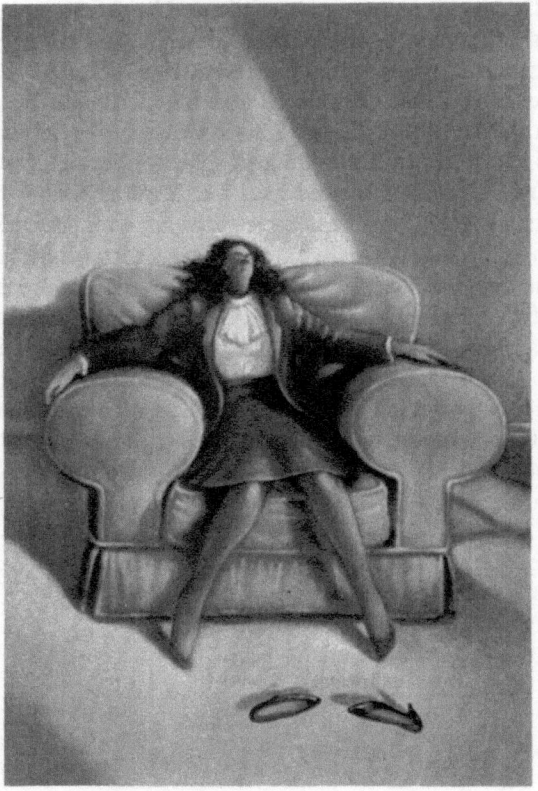

Figure 9.6 A typical 'fibromyalgia' patient (courtesy of Prof. R. Bennett)

Progress and management

Over the next 2–3 years the patient was hospitalized on several occasions in the UK, USA and Italy. She fell under the care of neurologists, rheumatologists, allergists and psychiatrists. She complained bitterly and persistently of severe pain and stiffness in the neck and shoulders particularly, as well as the low back.

The costs of her medical care over this period amounted to over £400 000. The disruption to her family (she has two children) and to her social life was devastating. She was treated with every known non-steroidal anti-inflammatory drug, pulse methylprednisolone (for suspected SLE), oral steroids, and methotrexate (for seronegative arthritis). During hospitalization in the USA, a diagnosis of fibrositis and pain augmentation syndrome was made and in the UK she was eventually diagnosed as fibromyalgia syndrome, with accompanying irritable bowel syndrome and sleep disturbance as well as subjective Sjögren's. Psychiatric treatment consisted of a variety of neuroleptics and antidepressants and included 22 shock treatments as well as attempts at hypnotherapy. A diagnosis of severe 'essential' hypochondriasis in an hysterical manipulative personality was made and the prognosis deemed hopeless.

Points for discussion

This highly instructive case demonstrates the frustration facing the clinician when confronted by a case of this nature. The severe muscle and joint pains prompted the institution of therapies such as parenteral steroids and methotrexate. This is symptomatic of the inability of most doctors to deal with severe fibromyalgia, particularly when accompanied by persistent psychogenic 'overlay'. Anxiety/depression and eventual hypochondriasis even, as in this patient, often accompany the condition and may not respond to any known or standard therapy.

The relationship of the condition to trauma, such as the CSF leak following myelography, is of interest, but unknown.

The association of muscular pain and 'spasm' with 'nodules', such as occurred in this patient, made the diagnosis possible after a number of years of negative investigations. The occurence of an irritable bowel syndrome, poor sleep and subjective complaints of dry eyes and/or mouth are typical. Tiredness or fatigue and other symptoms including headaches, subjective feelings of articular or periarticular or joint swellings, numbness and sciatica, a temporomandibular-joint syndrome and earache/toothache are also typical and occurred in our patient.

The danger of addiction to narcotics cannot be underemphasized and great care should be taken to avoid these at all costs. The differential diagnosis between this condition and psychogenic rheumatism, polymyalgia rheumatica in the elderly, polymyositis, hypothroidism and connective tissue diseases such as SLE, rheumatoid arthritis or ankylosing spondylitis is also clearly important.

Recent work has revealed an abnormal alpha pattern interrupting slow wave rhythm sleep on EEG (non-REM deep sleep), and electron microscopy does show changes in muscle fibres not visible on routine pathological studies.

Therapy suggested today is amitryptiline or Flexeril at night in an attempt to normalize sleep patterns. An exercise program which includes 'stretching' exercices and the use of heat may relieve symptoms. A minority of patients may, however, be made worse by exercise. Benefit may be obtained from non-straining exercise such as swimming. Non-steroidals are usually ineffective but salicylates may be useful. Injection of tender points with local analgesics or local steroids has been helpful and acupuncture has also been found to be effective. Other forms of therapy, such as TENS (transcutaneous electrical nerve stimulation) or biofeedback, may be of use in individual patients.

Comment

The treatment of this condition is unsatisfactory in many. It should always be considered in the differential diagnosis of the generalized 'aches and pains' syndrome. Most sufferers eventually have neurotic overlay and their management may even become psychologically difficult for the attending physicians.

References

1. Yunus M, Masi A T, Calabro J J et al. Primary fibromyalgia (fibrositis) clinical study of 50 patients with matched normal controls. Semin. Arthritis Rheum. 1981: 11, 151 – 171
2. Yunus M. Generalized fibromyalgia syndrome. In Euro Rheumatology (Athens, Greece). 1987: 231 – 234
3. Goldenburg D L. Fibromyalgia syndrome. An emerging but controversial condition. J. Am. Med. Assoc. 1987: 257, 2782 – 2787
4. Bennett R M. Fibromyalgia. J. Am. Med. Assoc. 1987: 257, 2082 – 2083
5. Bennett R M. The fibrositis syndrome. In Kelley E (ed.) Textbook of Rheumatology 3rd Edn. 1987, Philadelphia, W B Saunders

Appendix:
Commonly Used Tests in Rheumatology
and Abbreviations (where applicable)

1. HAEMATOLOGY			*Normal values*	*Units*
A. Blood Count				
Haemoglobin (Hb)	Male		15.5±2.5	g/dl
	Female		14 ± 2.5	
Haematocrit (PCV)	Male		0.47±0.07	g/dl
	Female		0.42±0.05	
Mean corpuscular volume (MCV)			85±8	fl
Mean corpuscular haemoglobin (MCH)			29.5±2.5	pg
Mean corpuscular haemoglobin concentration (MCHC)			33±2	g/dl
Leukocytes (WBC,WC)			4–11	$10^9/L$
Neutrophils (40–75%)			2.0–7.5	$10^9/L$
Lymphocytes (20–45%)			1.5–4.0	$10^9/L$
Monocytes (2–10%)			0.2–0.8	$10^9/L$
Eosinophils (1–6%)			0.04–0.4	$10^9/L$
Platelets			150–400	$10^9/L$
Reticulocytes			10–100	$10^9/L$

B. Serum Values		*Range of mean*	
Serum iron		12–26	mcmol/L
Total iron binding capacity (TIBC)		45–70	mcmol/L
Serum ferritin	Males	24–413	mcg/L
	Females	15–314	mcg/L
Serum B_{12}		>120	ng/L
Serum folate		2.5–20	mcg/L

C. Coagulation Tests

		Normal range	
Bleeding time		1–7	mins
Whole blood clotting time		<10	mins
Kaolin cephalin time (KCCT)		35–45	secs
Prothrombin time (PT)		10–14	secs
Partial thromboplastin time (PTT)		32–42	secs
Thrombin time		10–12	secs
Haptoglobin (as Hb binding capacity)		400–1700	mg/L
Fibrinogen degradation products (FDPs)		Absent/trace (<10 mg/L)	
Antithrombin III Antigenic	Males	0.20–0.33	g/L
	Females	0.19–0.32	g/L
Functional	Males	0.7–1.1	KU/L
	Females	0.6–1.1	KU/L
Euglobulin clot lysis time		>90	mins

2. IMMUNOLOGY

A. Immunoglobulins

IgG	6–15	g/L
IgH	0.45–1.5	g/L
IgA	0.9–3.3	g/L
C-reactive protein (CRP)	<10	mg/L

B. Immunohaematology

Cold agglutinin titre	<64

Complement (reported as g/L or %)

Third component (C3)	0.7–1.8	g/L
	60–140	%
Fourth component (C4)	0.16–0.45	g/L
	60–125	%
Second component (C2)	60–120	%
Alternative pathway	60–140	%
CH50	25–45	U/ml
	50–125	%

C1q	70–140	%
C11NHB	0.15–0.35	g/L
Immune complexes	<4.9	mg IgG/dl

C. Normal Values in Specific Rheumatological Tests:

Rheumatoid factor	*Normal value*
Latex screening	positive/negative
Latex test	< 1 in 20
Sheep cell agglutination test (Rose–Waaler)	< 1 in 32

Antinuclear antibodies conversions

1:40	25	U/ml
1:80	50	U/ml
1:160	100	U/ml
1:320	200	U/ml
1:640	400	U/ml
1:1280	800	U/ml
1:2560	1600	U/ml
1:10 000	6400	U/ml

Antibodies to DNA	< 10
(i) Farr assay	< 20% binding
(ii) Crithidia IFL assay	< 1 in 10

Organ specific antibodies	negative
gastric, parietal, adrenal, gonadal, pancreas (islet), salivary duct	(with neat serum)
Thyroid microsomes	< 1 in 10^2
Thyroglobulin	< 1 in 10

Non-specific organ antibodies	
Antinuclear	< 1 in 10
Mitochondrial	
Ribosomal	
Smooth muscle	< 1 in 40
Striated muscle	< 1 in 10
Liver/kidney microsomes	< 1 in 10

ENA
Sm, Ro, La, u1-RNP   negative

3. SERUM VALUES

A. General

		Normal range	Units
Total proteins		6.2 – 82	g/L
Albumin		36 – 52	g/L
Globulin		24 – 37	g/L
Sodium		135 – 145	mmol/L
Potassium		3.5 – 5	mmol/L
Chloride		98 – 108	mmol/L.
Bicarbonate		23 – 39	mmol/L
Calcium		2.3 – 2.7	mmol/L
Inorganic phosphate		0.8 – 1.4	mmol/L
Magnesium		0.7 – 0.95	mmol/L
Urea		3.3 – 8	mmol/L
Urate	Males	0.26 – 0.46	mmol/L
	Females	0.20 – 0.37	mmol/L
Creatinine		50 – 120	mcmol/L
Cholesterol		3.6 – 7.8	mmol/L
Triglycerides		<2.5	mmol/L
Glucose		2.5 – 4.7	mmol/L
Amylase		<300	U/L
Creatine clearance		70 – 140	ml/min
Plasma viscosity		1.5 – 1.72	cP

B. Liver Function Tests

Serum total bilirubin		5 – 17	mcmol/L
Serum alkaline phosphatase		30 – 130	IU/L
Serum aspartate aminotransferase (AST, SGOT)		5 – 40	IU/L
Serum alamine aminotransferase (ALT, SGPT)		10 – 40	IU/L
Serum gamma-glutamyl transpeptidase (GGT)	Males	<80	IU/L
	Females	<30	IU/L

202

C. Muscle Enzymes

Lactic dehydrogenase (LDH) *Total*		120 – 500	iu/L
Hydroxybutarate dehydrogenase (HBD) (cardiac isomer of LDH)		<140	iu/L
Creatinine phosphokinase	Males	<200	iu/L
(CPK, CK)	Females	<170	iu/L

4. CEREBROSPINAL FLUID

Total protein	0.2 – 0.4	g/L
Albumin	<0.4	g/L
IgG	<0.6	g/L
Glucose	70% of blood value	
	(2.4 – 4.5) mmol/L (2 h lag)	
Cell count		
WBCs	<5	10^6/L
RBCs	Nil	

5. URINE

Total protein	<150	mg/day
Albumin	<20	mg/L

REFERENCE

PRU Handbook of Clinical Immunochemistry: SAS Protein Reference Units A Milford Ward (ed.) PRU Publications, 1986

Index